ABC of

Ear, Nose and Throat

Fifth Edition

EDITED BY

Harold Ludman

Emeritus Consultant Surgeon in Otolaryngology, King's College Hospital, London, UK
Emeritus Consultant Surgeon in Neurotology, National Hospital for Neurology and Neurosurgery, London, UK

Patrick J Bradley

Consultant Head and Neck Oncologic Surgeon, Department of Otorhinolaryngology, Head and Neck Surgery, Queens Medical Centre, University of Nottingham, Nottingham, UK

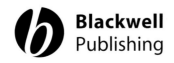

Blackwell Publishing

BMJ|Books

BMJ Books is an imprint of the BMJ Publishing Group Limited, used under licence

Blackwell Publishing, Inc., 350 Main Street, Malden, Massachusetts 02148-5020, USA
Blackwell Publishing Ltd, 9600 Garsington Road, Oxford OX4 2DQ, UK
Blackwell Publishing Asia Pty Ltd, 550 Swanston Street, Carlton, Victoria 3053, Australia

First published 1981
Second edition 1988
Third edition 1993
Fourth edition 1997
Fifth edition 2007

1 2007

Library of Congress Cataloging-in-Publication Data

ABC of ear, nose, and throat / edited by Harold Ludman and Patrick J. Bradley. -- 5th ed.
    p. ; cm.
  Rev. ed. of: ABC of otolaryngology / Harold Ludman. 1997.
  Includes bibliographical references and index.
  ISBN 978-1-4051-3656-3
  1. Otolaryngology. I. Ludman, Harold. II. Bradley, Patrick J., 1949-
III. Ludman, Harold. ABC of otolaryngology.
  [DNLM: 1. Otorhinolaryngologic Diseases. WV 140 A134 2007]

  RF46.A2344 2007
  617.5'1--dc22

                                         2006036143

ISBN: 978-1-4051-3656-3

A catalogue record for this title is available from the British Library

Cover image is courtesy of and adapted from University of Nebraska Medical Centre

Set in 9.25/12 pt Minion by Sparks, Oxford – www.sparks.co.uk
Printed and bound in Singapore by Fabulous Printers Pte Ltd

Associate Editor: Vicki Donald
Editorial Assistant: Victoria Pittman
Production Controller: Rachel Edwards

For further information on Blackwell Publishing, visit our website:
www.blackwellpublishing.com

Contents

Contributors

David Albert
Consultant Paediatric ENT Surgeon, Great Ormond Street Hospital, London, UK

Declan Costello
Specialist Registrar, John Radcliffe Hospital, Oxford, UK.

Kevin Gibbin
Consultant ENT Surgeon, Queens Medical Centre, Nottingham, UK

Nick S Jones
Consultant Rhinologist, Queens Medical Centre, Nottingham, UK

Julian McGlashan
Consultant ENT Surgeon, Queens Medical Centre, Nottingham, UK

William McKerrow
Consultant ENT Surgeon, Raigmore Hospital, Inverness, UK

Antony Narula
Consultant ENT Surgeon and Head of Department, St Mary's Hospital, London; Honorary Professor of Otolaryngology, Middlesex University, UK

Vinidh Paleri
Consultant Surgeon, Otolaryngology-Head and Neck Surgery, Newcastle upon Tyne University Hospitals, Newcastle, UK

Parag M Patel
Specialist Registrar, Royal Surrey County Hospital, Guildford, Surrey, UK

Shahed Quraishi
Consultant Head and Neck Surgeon, Doncaster Royal Infirmary, Doncaster, UK

Julian Rowe-Jones
Consultant Rhinologist and Nasal Plastic Surgeon, Guildford Nuffield Hospital, Guildford, Surrey, UK

Anshul Sama
Consultant Rhinolaryngologist, Queens Medical Centre, Nottingham, UK

Iain Swan
Consultant ENT Surgeon, Gartnavel General Hospital, Glasgow, UK

Archana Vats
Specialist Registrar, St Mary's Hospital, London, UK

Anthony Wright
Professor of Otolaryngology, Institute of Laryngology and Otology, University College London, London, UK

Preface to Fifth Edition

The first edition of this small volume, *The ABC of Ear, Nose and Throat*, was derived 25 years ago from a series of articles published at that time in the *British Medical Journal* to present the substance of this important speciality in an easily assimilable form for a wide readership of general practitioners, medical students, nurses and all those many sprouting paramedical specialties involved with speech, hearing, and head and neck disorders. This target readership has not changed, but the specialty, like most others, has expanded and developed subspecialties in all its divisions.

Otology has changed from the exciting renaissance of microscopic middle ear work that began in the 1960s at the start of my personal otological career, to the amazing developments that include cochlear implantation for inner ear deafness, and neuro-otology has extended from the management of peripheral labyrinthine disorders to embrace surgery within the base of the skull.

Rhinological change has brought us the endoscopic techniques that have revolutionized treatment for paranasal sinus diseases, while the management of throat malignancy has evolved out of all recognition into today's comprehensive management of head and neck tumours.

It is entirely appropriate therefore that, for this expanded fifth edition, Patrick Bradley FRCSIr, FRCSEd, FRCSEng, MBA, as an internationally recognized authority on head and neck diseases and their treatment, should have become the joint editor, and that several specialists, recognized as experts in various subspecialties, have been enlisted to write about them.

The title has appositely reverted to its briefer, earlier one of ENT, which is so quintessentially British and which trips much more readily off the tongue than does otolaryngology.

Harold Ludman

CHAPTER 1

Pain in the Ear

Harold Ludman

OVERVIEW

- Pain in the ear (otalgia) arises from:
  - acute inflammatory disease of the external ear or middle ear cleft;
  - diseases not primarily in the ear;
    - referral from other sites;
    - neurological disease;
    - psychogenic.

Pain is one of six symptoms that may indicate ear disease (Box 1.1). Inflammatory causes of pain are recognized by inspection of the external ear and tympanic membrane. An otoscope is usually used in general practice, but otologists always use a headlight or head mirror to provide vision coincident with the direction of illumination, allowing manipulation with freed hands and instruments for the removal of wax or debris, and for the assessment of drum mobility with a pneumatic speculum (Fig. 1.1).

A binocular microscope is invariably used for fine manipulation with micro instruments and suction apparatus for accurate assessment under magnification of six times or more (Fig. 1.2).

If the external ear canal and the tympanic membrane are *definitely* normal, then pain cannot arise from ear disease. The reliability of this judgement depends on the skill and experience of the examiner. A tympanic membrane may show subtle changes, which are not easily recognized, while some abnormalities are irrelevant. If in any doubt, an otological opinion should be sought (Fig. 1.3).

Box 1.1 **Symptoms of ear disease**

- pain
- discharge
- hearing loss
- tinnitus
- vertigo
- facial palsy

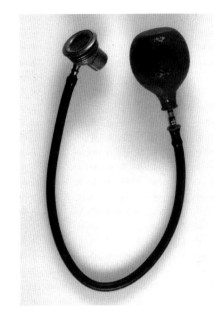

(a)

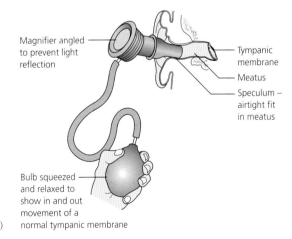

Magnifier angled to prevent light reflection

Tympanic membrane

Meatus

Speculum – airtight fit in meatus

Bulb squeezed and relaxed to show in and out movement of a normal tympanic membrane

(b)

Figure 1.1 (a) Photograph of pneumatic (Siegle's) speculum and (b) diagram showing its use.

Acute otitis externa

Acute otitis externa may be either diffuse – involving all the skin of the external meatus – or localized as a furuncle (Fig. 1.4).

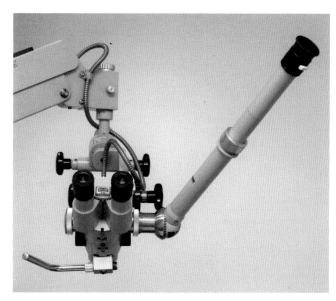

Figure 1.2 Binocular microscope with sidearm for observer.

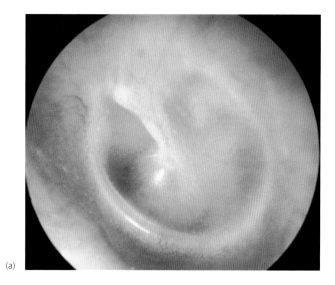

(a)

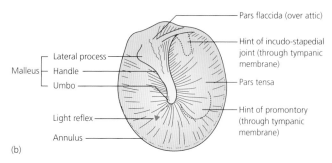

(b)

Figure 1.3 (a) Photograph of normal left tympanic membrane and (b) labelled diagram.

A furuncle is a very tender swelling (a boil). It is always in the outer ear canal, as there are no hair follicles in the inner bony meatus. Hearing is impaired only if the meatus becomes blocked by

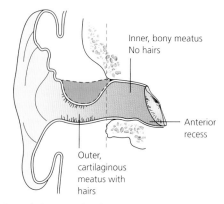

Figure 1.4 Furuncle in external auditory meatus.

swelling or discharge, and fever occurs only if infection spreads in front of the ear, as cellulitis or erysipelas. Superficially tender enlarged nodes may be palpable in front of or behind the ear. The pinna is tender to movement in acute otitis externa, but this is not the case in acute otitis media. Discharge, if any, is usually thick and scanty, unlike the copious mucoid discharge through tympanic membrane perforation from acute middle ear infections. Fungal skin infections cause severe pain with wet keratin desquamation and black or coloured granules of the fruiting heads of conidiophores.

Treatment of acute otitis externa

Systemic antibiotics are advised in acute otitis externa only if there is fever or lymphadenitis. Sometimes, meatal swelling must be reduced by inserting a ribbon gauze wick painted with a deliquescent substance such as magnesium sulphate paste, or glycerine and 10% ichthammol (Fig. 1.5). Proprietary 'Pope' wicks (Xomed) are thin and stiff to enable careful insertion, and they then soften and swell gently when moistened with liquid medication. A wick should be replaced daily until skin swelling subsides. Ear drops may then be used – either aluminium acetate to 'toughen' the skin or topical antibiotics, such as gentamicin, framycetin or neomycin, combined with steroids. Topical clotrimazole is a useful antifungal agent. Systemic analgesics, together with warmth, applied through a hot pad or heat lamp, relieve pain. Recurrent furunculosis should raise a suspicion of diabetes.

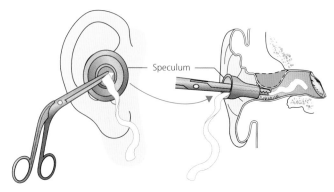

Figure 1.5 Inserting a wick.

Acute suppurative otitis media

Acute suppurative otitis media causes deep-seated pain, impaired hearing and systemic illness with fever. A blocked feeling in the ear then pain and fever, are followed by discharge if the tympanic membrane perforates – with relief of pain. The whole middle ear cleft is affected. This is the entire air-containing space comprising the Eustachian tube, the middle ear cavity, the mastoid antrum and its adjacent mastoid air cells (Fig. 1.6). For this reason, deep pressure over the mastoid antrum elicits tenderness in acute otitis media; this does not imply the development of mastoiditis. Bacterial infection is usually by *Streptococcus pneumoniae*, or *Haemophilus influenzae* in very young children. Diagnosis is made by inspecting the tympanic membrane, but this may be prevented by wax, or by swelling from a secondary otitis externa. *Only if the whole drum can be certified as normal and there is no conductive hearing loss* (demonstrated by tuning fork tests) can otitis media confidently be excluded. Adjacent lymph nodes are never enlarged in simple otitis media.

Treatment of acute suppurative otitis media

Systemic antibiotics are recommended. The commonest infecting organisms are *Streptococcus pneumoniae*, *Haemophilus influenzae* and *Moraxella (Branhamella) catarrhalis*. The antibiotic of choice, effective against all these, is amoxycillin. If β lactamase-producing organisms are likely, amoxycillin combined with clavulanic acid (Augmentin) or trimethoprin and sulphamethoxazole may be preferred. Oral administration is advised, even for the first dose, and medication must be continued for at least 5 days. Supplementary treatment includes pain relief by analgesics and warmth. Warm olive oil drops are soothing. If the tympanic membrane perforates, the ensuing discharge should be cultured, but an antibiotic should be changed on clinical and not bacteriological grounds. Rarely, the drum may bulge under pressure without rupture, requiring urgent incision to release pus (myringotomy).

Recurrent acute otitis media may be provoked by predisposing causes, such as persisting middle ear effusions, when a potentially infected accumulation of mucus persists in the middle ear cleft. Myringotomy with insertion of a ventilation tube or 'grommet' may then be advisable. Adenoid enlargement with repeated infection is probably also a causative factor, but the role of adenoidectomy remains controversial. In the absence of predisposing factors, each attack should be treated as it arises. After any episode, return to normal is expected and should be confirmed within 3 weeks.

Acute (coalescent) mastoiditis

Acute mastoiditis is caused by the breakdown of the thin bony partitions (trabeculae) between the mastoid air cells, which then become coalescent (Fig. 1.7). This process takes 2–3 weeks to occur fully. Throughout that time, there is, in most cases, continuing and increasingly copious discharge through a perforation in the drum, with general malaise and fever, unless this has been suppressed by antibiotics. If a patient has pain a few days after the tympanic membrane has been reliably judged to be normal, then that patient *cannot* have developed mastoiditis. Difficulties arise when a patient is thought to have recovered from acute otitis media, but in reality the condition has 'grumbled on', perhaps by suppression of systemic effects with antibiotics. Mastoiditis *should* be suspected in any patient with continuous discharge from the middle ear for over 10 days, particularly if he or she is continually unwell.

Radiographs or, better, CT scans of the mastoid air cells may help to diagnose the condition, but not always. Only if they show a clearly aerated normal cell system (Fig. 1.8) can mastoiditis be excluded. The classical appearance of breakdown of intracellular trabeculae is not always apparent. Otitis externa may cause apparent haziness of the air cell system because of oedema of the soft tissues over the mastoid process. The often-described traditional classical sign of a swelling behind the ear with downward displacement of the pinna implies a subperiosteal abscess. This is a complication rather than a feature of mastoiditis. A subperiosteal abscess can also, by erosion of the bony outer attic wall, cause swelling in the roof of the deep part of the external ear canal, in contrast with a furuncle, which arises only in its outer part. If any doubt persists after mastoid imaging, surgical exploration is advisable.

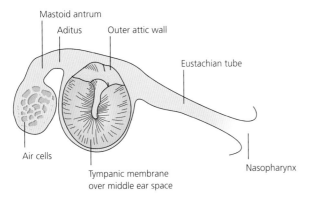

Figure 1.6 The middle ear cleft.

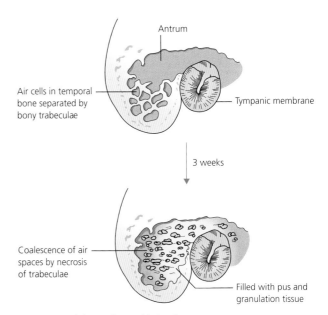

Figure 1.7 Breakdown of mastoid air cells.

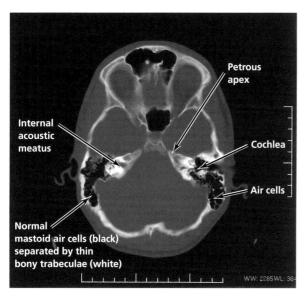

Figure 1.8 CT scan of normal mastoid air cells.

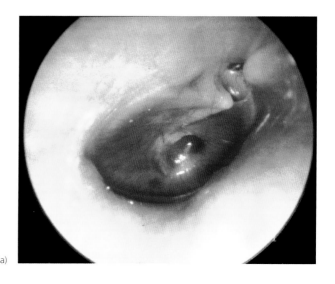

(a)

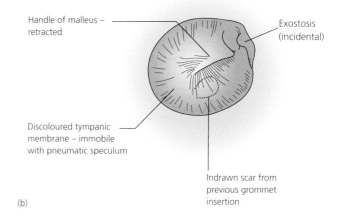

(b)

Figure 1.10 (a) Photograph of tympanic membrane with 'glue ear' and (b) labelled diagram.

Other complications of acute suppurative otitis media

These are all also possible complications of the bone erosive forms of chronic suppurative otitis media (see Chapter 2 and Fig. 1.9). They arise if infection spreads beyond the middle ear cleft itself. Complications occurring *within the petrous temporal bone* include facial palsy, suppurative labyrinthitis and lateral sinus thrombophlebitis; *those occurring within the cranial cavity* are meningitis, extradural abscess, subdural abscess and brain abscess (in the temporal lobe or cerebellum).

Chronic secretory otitis media (otitis media with effusion)

Niggly, short-lived pain is a common feature of 'glue ear'. The drum looks abnormal because of the effusion (Fig. 1.10). Classically, there is injection with visible radial vessels, which may prompt a misdiagnosis of otitis media. The colour may be yellowish or sometimes blue. The child is well and afebrile, however, and the associated hearing loss has usually been recognized for some time.

An essential diagnostic feature, which can be elicited by an otologist using a headlight and a pneumatic speculum, is altered mobility of the tympanic membrane. It may be totally immobile when external ear canal air pressure is raised and reduced, or there may be sluggish outward movement followed by a rapid 'snap' back when the partial vacuum is released. This altered mobility can also be demonstrated by tympanometry using an impedance measuring meter during continuously changing ear canal pressure – from above to below normal atmospheric level. Simple, automatic tympanometers print out a quickly available chart indicating middle ear air pressure and its changes (if any) as the external ear air pressure is raised and then lowered. However, there can be technical problems in using these devices reliably.

'Malignant' otitis externa

This is a rare but serious form of infection (not neoplastic, despite the name), caused by *Pseudomonas aeruginosa*, arising usually in elderly diabetics. It should be suspected if patients in this group

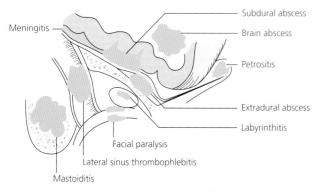

Figure 1.9 Complications of suppurative otitis media.

suffer severe pain, excessive for the signs of otitis externa. Infection invades the bony base of the skull and adjacent soft tissues. Facial paralysis and other cranial nerve palsies may develop, and mortality used to be high. A suspicious finding is granulation tissue in the ear canal, which must be investigated by CT scanning. Treatment with intravenous gentamicin, or with oral ciprofloxacin, is administered continuously for several weeks, and must not cease before recovery from pain.

Other causes of pain

Bullous myringitis is another cause of severe pain. Viral (probably influenzal) infection causes haemorrhagic blistering of the ear drum and external ear canal. There is often an associated haemorrhagic effusion in the middle ear and it may be difficult to distinguish this condition from otitis media. For that reason alone antibiotics may be administered, but the only necessary treatment is potent analgesia.

Referred pain

If the external ear canal and drum are normal, with normal movement of the drum on examination with a pneumatic speculum, pain cannot be due to disease of the ear. It may well be referred from territory sharing its ultimate sensory innervation with the outer or middle ear (Fig. 1.11). Pain therefore may arise from:

(a) The oropharynx (IXth nerve) in tonsillitis or carcinoma of the posterior third of the tongue.
(b) The laryngopharynx (Xth nerve) in carcinoma of the pyriform fossa.
(c) Upper molar teeth, temporomandibular joint or parotid gland (Vth nerve mandibular division). Parotid causes are usually obvious: impacted wisdom teeth may not be. Temporomandibular joint troubles often follow changes in bite caused by new dentures, extraction or grinding down.
(d) The cervical spine (C2 and C3). Pain is often worse at night when the head lies awkwardly. Neck support often provides relief, as does a neck pillow under the side of the neck during sleep.

If there is no inflammatory ear disease and no disease in sites from which pain might be referred to the ear, remaining possibilities include glossopharyngeal neuralgia, migrainous neuralgia or psychogenic pain.

Often no cause can be found; it may sometimes be attributed to depression and a trial of antidepressive medication can be advised.

Further reading

Kerr A, Booth J. (eds) (1997) *Scott Brown's Otolaryngology, 6th Edition*. Butterworth-Heinemann, Oxford.
Ludman H, Wright T. (eds) (1998) *Diseases of the Ear, 6th Edition*. Arnold-Hodder Headline, London.

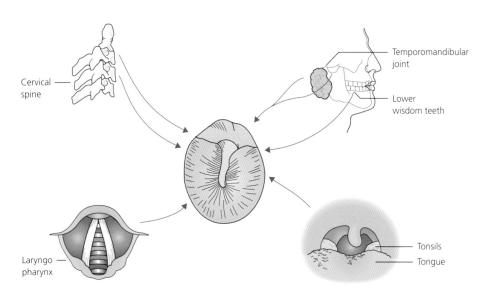

Figure 1.11 Origins of referred pain.

CHAPTER 2

Discharge from the Ear

Harold Ludman

OVERVIEW

Aural discharge arises from:

- acute suppurative otitis media (and a subacute continuation);
- chronic suppurative otitis media, in one of two forms: 'safe' and 'unsafe';
- chronic otitis externa (and as a feature of acute otitis externa);
- very rarely as cerebrospinal fluid after head injury.

Discharge from the ear (otorrhoea) can suggest acute otitis externa or otitis media, and is usually the main feature of chronic inflammatory diseases of the external ear or middle ear (Box 2.1 and Fig. 2.1).

In acute disease, pain invariably dominates and precedes discharge (see Chapter 1).

Acute otitis media

Acute suppurative otitis media produces profuse mucopurulent or purulent discharge after the pain, if the drum perforates. As the perforation heals, the discharge ceases.

Box 2.1 **Source of discharge must be identified by full otological examination**

- Tympanic membrane (TM) intact and normal = otitis externa
- TM with perforation = otitis media

Increasingly profuse discharge persisting for more than 10 days may suggest acute coalescent mastoiditis, especially if the patient is febrile with deep tenderness over the mastoid antrum, behind the pinna (see Chapter 1).

'Subacute' suppurative otitis media

Now that acute mastoiditis is rare, a common syndrome is that of a 'well' child continuously discharging mucopus from the ear for three or more weeks after a typical attack of acute suppurative otitis media. Often, grommets have been sited in the ear drum. Continuing mucosal infection of the middle ear by resistant organisms, continuing infection of the nasopharynx with secondary infection of the middle ear cleft, and changes in the mucosa of the middle ear secondary to Eustachian tube dysfunction may all contribute. A grommet may be irritating the adjacent tissues, suggested by adjacent granulation tissue visible to inspection, around its edges on the surface of the tympanic membrane.

Swab culture will indicate appropriate antibiotics to give systemically. After regular gentle toilet to remove infected debris from the meatus, topical antibiotic and steroid drops should be massaged into the middle ear by pressure on the tragus, for 5–7 days (Fig. 2.2).

Children should learn to blow their noses to prevent mucus stagnation with infection. Decongestant nasal sprays may help, after blowing the nose, for a short period only – up to a week. Systemic antihis-

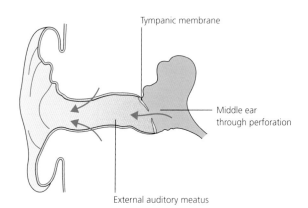

Figure 2.1 Where does discharge come from?

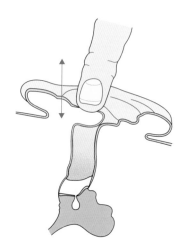

Figure 2.2 Massaging drops into the middle ear.

tamines may also be part of the regimen, to reduce allergic swelling of the mucosa around the orifice of the Eustachian tube. Provided mastoiditis can be excluded, these measures can be used without fear of serious risk for several weeks. If the discharge continues, referral is recommended, when removal of enlarged adenoids may be advised. Sometimes, enlarging a small perforation in the tympanic membrane under general anaesthetic (GA) improves the condition and provides an opportunity for suction removal of material from the middle ear. An irritating grommet suggested by granulation tissue should be removed under GA.

Rarely, continuing discharge may suggest that the mucosa throughout the mastoid air cell system has become muco-secretory in nature. This may be an indication for a cortical mastoidectomy.

Chronic otitis externa

The discharge is usually accompanied by itching and irritation. It is often thick and smelly, from infected wax and desquamating skin. The organisms are usually Gram negative. The ear drum, when exposed, is found to be normal, and there is no hearing loss. Examination of the drum head can be difficult because of meatal swelling and debris within it. Suction removal of dead material is needed, using a microscope, with particular attention to the anterior recess, where the meatus curves forward to make an acute angle with the drum beyond.

Chronic otitis externa is partly due to skin diseases – eczema, seborrhoeic dermatitis or psoriasis – and partly to external trauma to the ears from wetting, drying with a dirty towel or scratching.

Chronic otitis externa is treated by so-called aural toilet and the application of topical medication. Cleaning to remove infected debris must be performed under good illumination, using cotton wool on a wire wool carrier, or by suction under a microscope.

Toilet should be repeated, ideally every day. Microbial swabs for fungi as well as bacteria will guide the choice of topical applications, such as combinations of antibiotics like gentamicin and neomycin with a steroid. Fungal infections need antifungal agents such as nystatin or clotrimazole. Medication may be instilled as drops twice a day, painted on the meatal walls with cotton wool on a wire wool carrier, inserted on an impregnated gauze wick, or insufflated as a powder after toilet. Eczematous reactions of the pinna require application of antiallergic creams or ointments (Fig. 2.3).

Systemic antibiotics are never necessary. Topical preparations should not be used for long periods (7–10 days at most). There is, however, a case for applying drops intermittently (for example once a week) to try to prevent repeated relapses.

When intrinsic factors predominate, permanent cure rather than alleviation may be impossible. Subepithelial fibrosis can cause gross narrowing of the meatus, causing lack of ventilation and difficulties in performing adequate toilet. An operation to widen the meatus is then needed. All patients who have had chronic otitis externa must be warned to protect their ears from water and never poke cotton buds or other implements into the meatus.

Chronic suppurative otitis media

There are two forms of chronic suppurative otitis media, which should be considered as distinct and separate entities. Both present

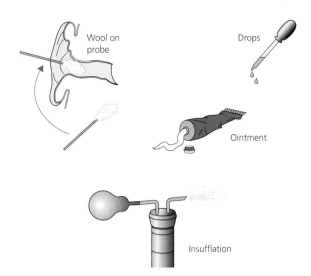

Figure 2.3 Applying medication to the external auditory meatus.

with conductive deafness and discharge without pain. In both, discharge issues through a perforated drum; however, one is styled 'safe', while the other is 'unsafe', because of potentially serious complications (Fig. 2.4).

The **safe variety** (or active mucosal chronic otitis media) carries no serious risks. Disease affects the mucosa of the lower front part of the middle ear cleft ('tubotympanic'). In contrast, the **unsafe variety** (active chronic with cholesteatoma) threatens the hazard of spread of infection intracranially. This disease is associated with erosion of surrounding bone. Cholesteatoma (described below) or chronic osteitis involves the upper back part of the middle ear cleft, and so anatomically it is described as 'atticoantral'.

In the safe type, the perforation is 'central' (Fig. 2.5). By this, it is meant that no matter how large the defect, there is always a rim of drum or even just its annulus around the edge. It involves the vibrating part of the tympanic membrane – the pars tensa, below the malleolar folds, at the level of the lateral process of the malleus.

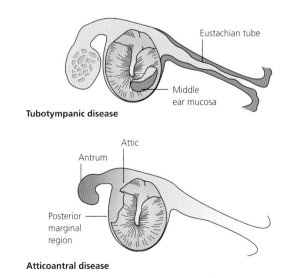

Figure 2.4 Two types of chronic suppurative otitis media.

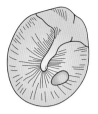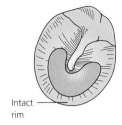

Intact
rim

Figure 2.5 Central perforations.

The perforation in the unsafe variety extends into the very bony edge of the drum, where it produces chronic bone necrosis and is associated with the production of granulation tissue or a polyp. This so-called marginal perforation (Fig. 2.6) is usually posterior, or in the attic region of the drum head above the malleolar folds – the pars flaccida.

Discharge from the 'safe' variety arises from the inflamed and secreting mucosa of the middle ear and is copious, mucoid or mucopurulent. It may be intermittent. In the 'unsafe' variety the discharge is scanty, foul smelling and continuous. It comes from infected debris accumulating within a *cholesteatoma sac* (Fig. 2.7). Cholesteatoma is skin – stratified squamous keratinizing epithelium – that has invaded the middle ear cleft to form a cyst surrounding the ossicular contents of the attic, descending into the middle ear mesotympanum and extending back into the mastoid antrum and its connecting air cells. When the accumulating keratin within the cholesteatoma becomes infected, its outermost layer, which is the basal layer of the skin, develops a propensity to erode adjacent bone, threatening spread of infection beyond.

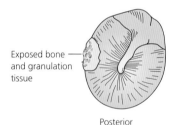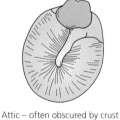

Exposed bone
and granulation
tissue

Posterior   Attic – often obscured by crust

Figure 2.6 Marginal perforations.

Recognition and treatment of safe ears

The distinction between the two kinds of chronic suppurative otitis media is made by examining the ear drum after removing any discharge – ideally under an operating microscope and sometimes under anaesthetic. It is often impossible to make a certain and reliable distinction on a first inspection.

In safe ears, the aim is to eliminate discharge and possibly to assist hearing deficit. Drying is achieved by treating infection or allergy in the upper respiratory tract and by aural toilet to remove infected material. Antibiotic drops containing steroids are routinely useful.

Once the ear is dry, the state may be described as 'inactive chronic otitis media', and recurrent discharge may often be prevented by protecting the ear from water and by promptly treating upper respiratory tract infection, or by closing the defect in the ear drum surgically (myringoplasty). Hearing defects may, if necessary, be helped by using a hearing aid, or by reconstructing the drum and the ossicular chain (tympanoplasty).

Treatment of unsafe ears

An unsafe ear must be rendered harmless as the priority before considering tackling any hearing loss. The traditional approach is to remove diseased and infected bone and to fashion a smooth, wide cavity opening into a wide external ear canal. As the ear heals, the cavity becomes lined with skin, which is histologically identical to cholesteatoma but which excretes its dead squames easily to the exterior through wide access to the external ear canal. Operations are named according to the extent of bone removal, which is dictated by the extent of disease.

Radical mastoidectomy is one extreme of this kind of operation. The mastoid antrum is opened with a drill. As access to the antrum is enlarged, it is extended forward into the attic region of the middle ear. Removal of bone over the attic and antrum joins the mastoid cavity and middle ear into one. Diseased material is extirpated as the operation proceeds. All the ossicular chain except the stapes is removed. The cavity is made as hemispherical as possible, while respecting the safety of the adjacent facial nerve, labyrinth, sigmoid sinus and dura (Fig. 2.8). Lesser cavity operations, dictated by the disease limits, are called atticotomy, attico-antrostomy or modified radical mastoidectomy, depending on their extent. Parts of the ossicular chain and tympanic membrane may safely be preserved.

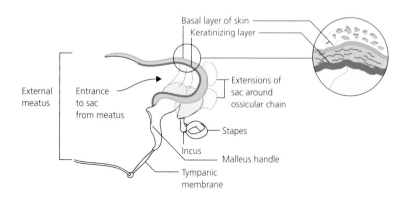

Basal layer of skin
Keratinizing layer

External
meatus

Entrance
to sac
from meatus

Extensions of
sac around
ossicular chain

Stapes

Incus

Malleus handle

Tympanic
membrane

Figure 2.7 Cholesteatoma
sac in attic.

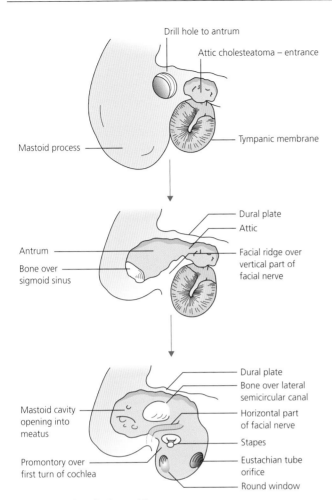

Figure 2.8 Right radical mastoidectomy.

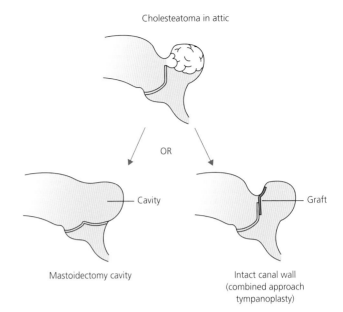

Figure 2.9 Two strategies for treating unsafe ears.

All of these 'open cavity' operations are liable to repeated discharge, which may be provoked if their lining is exposed to ingress of water. Therefore swimming is to be avoided.

Alternatives include so-called combined approach tympanoplasty, or intact canal wall techniques, which aim to avoid cavity creation and include attempts to reconstruct the middle ear mechanism (Fig. 2.9). They entail a risk of enclosing residual cholesteatoma, but avoid repeated or continuous discharge and aim to preserve hearing and offer safe swimming. The possibility of residual cholesteatoma skin demands repeated operations essential for its discovery and removal every year or two until no skin or so-called 'epithelial pearls' are discovered. This may need two or three subsequent procedures, and limits the application of these techniques to reliable patients who will not go absent from continuing care. However, after such closed operations, swimming can safely be resumed.

The dangerous complications of unsafe ears, excluding acute mastoiditis that occurs only after acute infection, are all listed in Chapter 1. It is beyond the scope of this work to consider these in detail, but suffice it to say that any patient with a discharging middle ear who complains of headache, vertigo or facial weakness must be referred urgently for expert evaluation.

Discharge from a mastoid cavity

After open cavity operations, discharge continues until the cavity becomes completely lined with skin, a process that usually takes 3 months and in some patients is never complete. Continuing or recurrent discharge arises from anything that prevents or breaks down an intact cavity lining. A warm, damp, mastoid cavity is inhospitable to healthy skin. Conditions for healing are best when operation creates as small a cavity with as wide an opening into the external meatus as feasible. Discharge becomes infected with Gram-negative organisms from outside (water), or from the nasopharynx. Infected material deters skin healing. Granulations that cannot be covered by epithelium may develop to occlude poorly drained pockets of infected material. Rarer causes of continuing discharge include residual bone disease and metaplasia of the normal mastoid cavity lining to mucus secreting epithelium.

During the early postoperative period, the ear, protected by a gauze pad or cotton wool, is left to heal. Water must not get in. Later, if there is surface infection, gentle cleaning and treatment with topical antibiotics and steroids, or boric acid powder, are used. Treatment of hearing loss after an ear has been rendered safe depends on the state of the other ear. Options include use of a hearing aid, or reconstructive surgery (tympanoplasty).

Further reading

Kerr A, Booth J. (eds) (1997) *Scott Brown's Otolaryngology, 6th Edition*. Butterworth-Heinemann, Oxford.

Ludman H, Wright T. (eds) (1998) *Diseases of the Ear, 6th Edition*. Arnold-Hodder Headline, London.

CHAPTER 3

Hearing Impairment and Tinnitus in Adults

Harold Ludman

OVERVIEW

The effects and causes of hearing impairment in adults, and their correction, are discussed, including:

- the distinction between conductive and sensorineural deafness;
- the recognition of these, and their causes;
- the assessment of hearing loss and its diagnostic causes;
- the correction of conductive defects;
- current views on the management of tinnitus.

(Assistance for deafness that cannot be corrected is discussed in Chapter 4.)

Box 3.1 **Effects**

These affect the effects of hearing loss:

- severity;
- age of onset;
- rate of onset;
- unilateral or bilateral.

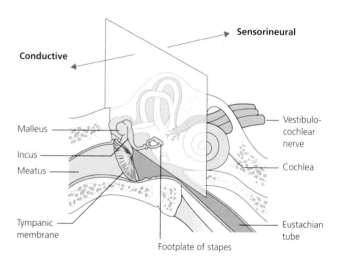

Figure 3.1 Distinction between conductive and sensorineural hearing loss.

The effects of hearing impairment depend on the severity of loss, the rate of onset, whether one or both ears are affected and the age of onset (Box 3.1). A baby born deaf in both ears cannot learn to speak without special help and normal language development will be impossible if the deafness is severe. A child with good speech will almost certainly lose it if severely deafened in the first years of life. An adult who becomes very deaf does not lose vocabulary, but the lack of auditory feedback degrades the voice into a harsh flat monotone. Rapid total deafness in both ears is a catastrophe that affects every aspect of the victim's life, whereas gradually developing loss causes serious but less severe handicap. By comparison, total loss of hearing in one ear is relatively trivial, regardless of age.

Deafness is one of the cruellest forms of sensory deprivation. Unlike blindness, it often provokes ridicule rather than sympathy and understanding. Unable to hear what is said, and unable to control his or her own voice, the severely deaf person may appear to others to be distracted and disengaged at best, mentally deficient at worst. Isolated from family and friends and greeted by unsympathetic attitudes, he or she often becomes depressed. Tinnitus, which often accompanies deafness and is rarely found without it, can cause distress as great as that from lack of hearing.

The prevalence of hearing loss is not accurately known: probably over 3 million adults (6 in every 100 in the UK) have impaired hearing and over 10 000 children need special education.

The two main types of defect are conductive and sensorineural. Hearing defects are described as *conductive* when there is impediment to the passage of sound waves between the external ear and the footplate of the stapes, or *sensorineural* if there is a fault in the cochlea (sensory), or the cochlear nerve (neural) (Fig. 3.1).

Conductive deafness

There are five possible mechanical faults that cause conductive deafness, outlined below.

Obstruction of the external ear canal

This is most commonly by wax, but can be from inflammatory oedema of the ear canal skin or accumulation of debris and discharge in the meatus. Less common causes are atresia, which can be congenital, and foreign bodies (Fig. 3.2a).

Perforation of the tympanic membrane

Sound transmission is affected by the reduced surface area of the drum for reception of incident sound waves, by admitting pressure waves to the middle ear to act adversely on the inner drum surface

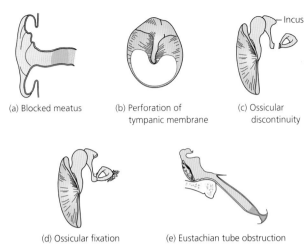

(a) Blocked meatus

(b) Perforation of tympanic membrane

(c) Ossicular discontinuity

(d) Ossicular fixation

(e) Eustachian tube obstruction

Figure 3.2 Common reasons for conductive deafness. (a) Blocked meatus; (b) perforation of tympanic membrane; (c) ossicular discontinuity; (d) ossicular fixation and (e) eustachian tube obstruction.

or by exposing the round window to incident sound pressure, which counters the normal cochlear endolymphatic wave effects.

Perforations can follow infective damage or trauma, especially by blows from the flat of a hand. They also more rarely follow sudden diving pressure changes (Fig. 3.2b).

Discontinuity of the ossicular chain

This is usually subsequent to infective damage. In particular, the long process of the incus is often eroded. Dislocation may follow closed head injuries, with or without skull fracture (Fig. 3.2c).

Fixation of the ossicular chain

This is the characteristic feature of otosclerosis. This inherited disorder progressively immobilizes the footplate of the stapes in the oval window. No other part of the ossicular chain is ever affected. Otosclerosis must not be confused with tympanosclerosis, in which hyaline material is deposited under the mucosa of any part of the middle ear cleft, after repeated episodes of inflammation. These deposits may often be seen as 'chalk patches' in the ear drum and may restrict movement in any part of the chain (Fig. 3.2d).

Eustachian tube inadequacy

Incomplete or defective Eustachian tube function is very common in children and is accompanied by accumulation of extremely viscous material or effusion in the middle ear – so-called glue ear. Air is absorbed from the middle ear cleft, the tympanic membrane is pushed inwards by outside air pressure impairing free vibration, and fluid then accumulates within the middle ear air space. Glue ear is the commonest cause of acquired deafness in children of school age. Apart from faults in the maturation of normal tube opening, the nasopharyngeal orifice of the tube may be obstructed. The role of enlarged and repeatedly infected adenoids in preventing ventilation of the middle ear is controversial. Effusions in an adult middle ear are usually thin and serous. Although they often follow upper respiratory tract viral infections or barotrauma during aircraft de-

scent, carcinoma of the nasopharynx must be excluded as it may present with a conductive deafness from a middle ear effusion (Fig. 3.2e and 5.9).

Sensorineural deafness

Three main patterns of sensorineural deafness are recognized.

Bilateral progressive loss

This is usually from degenerative ageing changes in the cochlea – presbyacusis. Other important causes are drug ototoxicity and noise damage. Ototoxic drugs include the aminoglycoside antibiotics, especially when used systemically. Risks are greater in the elderly and those with impaired renal function. Irreversible damage may continue after treatment ceases. Drug blood levels must be regularly monitored during treatment.

Excessive noise damages the hair cells of the organ of Corti. This may follow brief high-intensity exposure (acoustic trauma), but is usually caused by high-intensity exposure over long periods. Such noise-induced hearing loss is important in industry and is a hazard of noisy leisure activities such as shooting and using power tools. The severity of damage depends on the intensity of the noise, duration of exposure and individual susceptibility.

Unilateral progressive sensorineural loss

This always suggests a form of Menière's disease (endolymphatic hydrops), or an acoustic neuroma (see Box 3.2), which must be excluded by investigation (below).

Sudden sensorineural deafness

This condition, fortunately, is usually unilateral. One cause is trauma to the head or ear; if there is a leak of perilymph from the oval or round window membranes, this may be surgically corrected. Other causes include viral infections (particularly mumps, measles and varicella zoster) or sudden impairment of cochlear blood flow. Sudden hearing loss may also announce the presence of an acoustic neuroma. Barotrauma from scuba diving may cause perilymph leakage into the middle ear, and reqires hospital admission for serial audiometry and possible tympanotomy.

Syphilis should also be considered with any of the patterns of acquired sensorineural hearing loss. Serological investigations are essential whenever another reasonable explanation is lacking.

Assessment

Full assessment of hearing loss demands the specification, for each ear, of the site of the defect, the cause, the severity of disability and handicap. When these can be stated, which is not always possible,

---

Box 3.2 **Acoustic neuroma suspicion**

Suspect an acoustic neuroma and refer to otologist whenever sensorineural loss is:
• Unilateral progressive
• Unilateral of sudden onset.

an attempt can then be made to determine (a) whether the defect is treatable with a possibility of improving hearing, (b) the overall handicap to life in general, considering hearing in both ears and (c) whether the deafness is a symptom of another disease – for example, syphilis or acoustic neuroma.

Important aspects of the history include the rate of onset and progression, family history, any information about noise exposure or unusual medication and associated aural symptoms (pain, discharge, vertigo and tinnitus). Examination will show whether the external ear canal is obstructed and, if not, the state of the ear drum. Obstructing wax or debris must be removed. The otologist generally removes it manually under the illumination of a headlight using wax hooks and rings, or cotton wool on wire carriers, but the general practitioner may prefer to *syringe* wax from the ear. For safety, there should be no previous history of middle ear disease or suspicion of perforation. A story of previous uneventful syringing is always comforting. If the wax is hard, it may be softened by instilling olive oil or 5% sodium bicarbonate drops, twice a day, for a few days beforehand. Proprietary ceruminolytic drops should be used with great care as they may cause otitis externa with swelling of the meatal skin and severe pain if the canal is already filled with hard wax.

When the canal is clear, the drum can be examined – preferably with an otoscope and a pneumatic speculum to assess mobility. Without this manoeuvre, a middle ear effusion may be overlooked because the drum may look surprisingly normal even when the whole middle ear is filled with mucoid material. At this stage, an otologist will always examine the ear under a binocular operating microscope.

A conductive loss can be distinguished from a sensorineural one by the use of two tuning fork tests – the Rinne and the Weber. For each, the ideal fork has a frequency of 512 Hz (cycles per second).

Rinne test

The examiner first establishes that the vibrating fork is audible at the meatus and on the mastoid process. The foot of the vibrating fork is then pressed on the mastoid bone behind the ear under test. Then it is moved to the external meatus and the patient is asked whether it can still be heard. If so, the fork is returned to the mastoid and the question repeated. By alternating this manoeuvre the examiner can establish reliably where the fork is heard longer. When conductive mechanisms are normal (giving a positive Rinne, recorded as AC > BC), the test shows better (more prolonged) hearing by air conduction at the meatus. Positive responses are found in normal ears, as would be expected teleologically, and in those with a sensorineural hearing loss.

When the loss is conductive, bone conduction, where sound is transmitted directly to the cochlea through the skull, remains unimpaired, whereas the response to air-conducted sound is diminished. As the hearing loss increases, the sound is heard for longer by bone conduction than by air conduction. This is a *negative Rinne* (BC > AC). If, however, one ear is totally deaf while the other retains good hearing, bone-conducted sound from the deaf side will be heard undiminished through the skull by the intact cochlea on the other side, giving rise to a so-called *false negative Rinne*. To expose this false negative, the test should be repeated while a loud sound is introduced to 'mask' the normal ear – for example, with a Barany noise box.

A quicker way to carry out the Rinne test is to present the fork first by air conduction at the meatus, then by bone conduction on the mastoid process and to ask which stimulus seems louder (Fig. 3.3a).

Weber test

The foot of the vibrating fork is placed on the forehead and the patient is asked in which ear the sound is heard. This test is particularly useful when hearing is very different in the two ears. When the hearing defect is sensorineural, the fork will be lateralized to the better side. The reverse is obtained when the deafness is conductive, with the impaired ear apparently receiving the stimulus.

With a combination of conductive and sensorineural loss, the normally reliable results of tuning fork tests may be misleading (Fig. 3.3b).

Audiometric tests

Quantitative measures of the loss, and accurate determination of its site and cause, depend on audiometric tests.

The most familiar is pure tone threshold audiometry. Performed with electronic equipment (Fig. 3.4) and standardized techniques in a soundproofed room, this establishes the severity of the hearing loss throughout a range of frequencies from 250 to 8000 Hz. At each frequency, the hearing loss is measured and plotted on a logarithmic decibel scale, with reference to normal hearing at that frequency, to produce an air conduction audiogram. A bone conduction thresh-

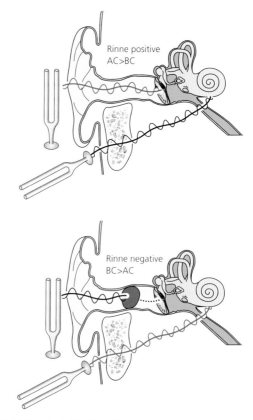

(a)

Figure 3.3 (a) Rinne test. (*Continued.*)

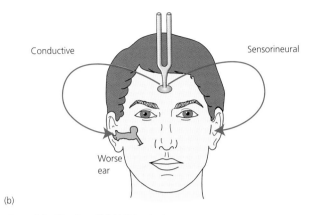

(b)

Figure 3.3 (*Continued.*) (b) Weber test.

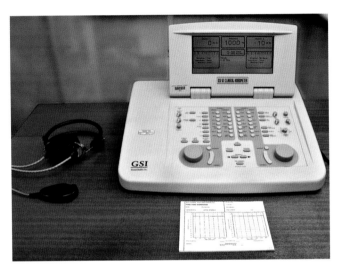

Figure 3.4 Pure tone audiometer.

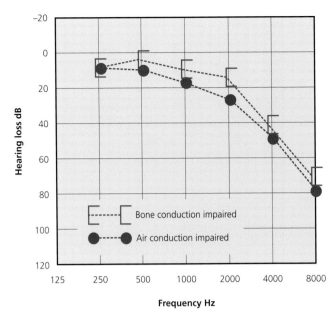

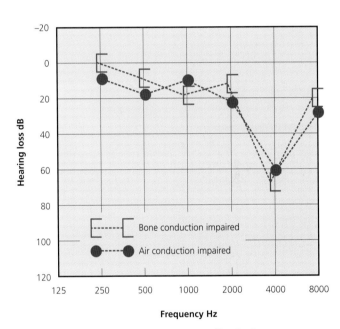

Figure 3.5 Pure tone audiogram in sensorineural hearing losses.

old audiogram can be produced by a transducer on the mastoid, with the untested ear masked against the test stimulus by the introduction of narrow-band white noise. By comparing the air and bone conduction thresholds, a 'quantified Rinne test' at different frequencies is available, allowing conductive and sensorineural hearing losses to be recognized. Bone conduction thresholds must be regarded with caution. They are less accurate and reliable than air conduction thresholds.

A pure tone audiogram provides some evidence of the type of hearing loss and indicates its severity. In some cases, the pattern of the curve suggests the cause (Figs 3.5 and 3.6).

More specialized tests in the outpatient clinic are needed to assess further the severity of the disability (although pure tone audiograms are surprisingly useful for this), but mainly to identify the site of the lesion.

Acoustic impedance measurements allow middle ear air pressure to be assessed by tympanometry and middle ear effusions (otitis media with effusion) to be recognized (Figs 5.5 and 5.6). This technique records contraction of the stapedius muscle in response to

auditory stimuli and is useful for recognizing conductive defects and in sensorineural diagnosis.

Speech audiometry examines discrimination ability above threshold. It measures the proportion of spoken words recognizable at different intensities and, by comparison with the pure tone audiogram, indicates whether a sensorineural defect lies in the cochlea or auditory nerve. Tests for so-called 'loudness recruitment' and 'adaptation' have a venerable history, but their discussion is beyond the scope of this work. *Brain stem electric response audiometry* is now the technique of choice for making the distinction between sensory and neural lesions. This is the standard audiometric test used whenever

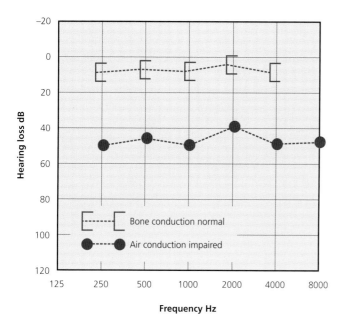

Figure 3.6 Pure tone audiogram in conductive hearing loss – bone conduction normal, air conduction impaired.

an acoustic neuroma is suspected, with high specificity and sensitivity. Final diagnosis of an acoustic neuroma nowadays entails enhanced magnetic resonance imaging (see Chapter 6).

Management

Helping patients with uncorrectable hearing defects, which include most instances of sensorineural loss, is discussed in Chapter 4. What can be done to help one ear depends on the state of the other. Theoretically, most conductive defects can be remedied.

Stapedectomy is used in otosclerosis (Fig. 3.7). It has led to the development of microsurgery of the ear during the past 40–50 years. The disability caused by the immobile stapes footplate is relieved by replacing the stapes with a plastic (or metal) prosthesis attached laterally to the long process of the incus, transmitting pressure medially to the perilymph of the inner ear within the vestibule.

Perforated ear drums are repaired by *myringoplasty*. A graft, usually of connective tissue (such as temporalis fascia), is placed, usually on the inner surface of the drum, after it has been prepared by removing its surface layer (Fig. 3.8).

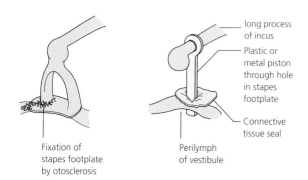

long process
of incus

Plastic or
metal piston
through hole
in stapes
footplate

Connective
tissue seal

Fixation of
stapes footplate
by otosclerosis

Perilymph
of vestibule

Figure 3.7 Stapedectomy (one technique).

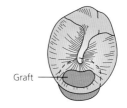

Graft

Figure 3.8 Underlay graft myringoplasty.

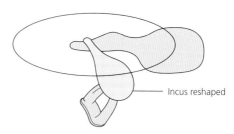

Incus reshaped

Figure 3.9 One form of ossiculoplasty with modified incus.

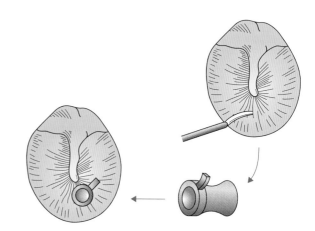

Figure 3.10 Insertion of grommet.

Breaks in the ossicular chain are repaired by various reconstructions (*ossiculoplasties*) to attach the ossicles to each other (Fig. 3.9), using artificial materials, such as hydroxyl apatite, or ossicular bone. Rebuilding of both the ossicular chain and the defective drum is a *tympanoplasty*. (This term also describes reconstructive procedures during excision of diseased tissue.)

Secretory otitis media (otitis media with effusion) and glue ear are relieved by a myringotomy incision in the anterior ear drum, aspiration of the effusion, and insertion of a ventilation tube or *grommet* to ventilate the middle ear cleft (Figs 3.10 and 5.10). Different kinds of grommet stay in place for different lengths of time, and the choice depends on the otologist's intentions for the duration of external ventilation.

All operations on the ear carry risks of cochlear damage, particularly if the inner ear has to be opened as in stapedectomy.

Tinnitus

Many deaf patients find tinnitus as or more distressing than the hearing loss, while for perhaps 25% of patients not particularly troubled by hearing disability, or even unaware of it, tinnitus is a dominant problem. In conductive hearing loss, tinnitus may be the result of removing ambient noise so that bodily activities become audible. Tinnitus is called objective when it is created by sound generated within the body by vascular tumours, abnormal blood flow, or by palatal myoclonus.

All normal people experience tinnitus at times, and most do when in soundproofed surroundings. The current understanding of the neurophysiology of the symptom, developed over the past 20 years, emphasizes that the response to sound reaching the auditory cortex is determined by its emotional connotations, from the limbic system, and their effect on the autonomic nervous centres responsible for emergency responses to potentially threatening sounds. Resting random activity in the central auditory system is only just below that at which sound enters consciousness: this is the price paid for the sensitivity of normal hearing. It is not surprising, then, that neuronal activity may become audible when a peripheral auditory defect provokes enhanced sensitivity to sound by compensatory 'resetting'. This arises in sensorineural hearing impairment in an attempt to overcome the hearing deficit, and is responsible for the hyperacusis and lowered loudness discomfort levels that are closely associated with tinnitus. The effect of that awareness on the limbic and autonomic centres is now recognized as the source of the distress, or lack thereof, in the presence of neuronal activity responsible for tinnitus. The degree of suffering is unrelated to the characteristics of the tinnitus perception. No drugs, and certainly no operative measures, such as cochlear nerve section, are helpful in treating tinnitus. Indeed, nerve section is usually harmful in causing or exacerbating the symptom.

Management nowadays entails so-called *tinnitus retraining therapy* (TRT), using psychological techniques to alter the autonomic response to the emotional content of the auditory pathways. This form of management must be conducted by fully trained counsellors. The skills cannot be acquired without experience in a recognized and reputable practising TRT centre. The heart of the problem is to remove the negative feedback to the sound experience that continually enhances the distress it causes. In the absence of negative or positive feedback, perceived sound is ignored – and is free from autonomic distress provocation, as are the many environmental sounds we ignore daily – by the process called habituation. Initially, there must be a sensible explanation of the mechanism, accepted by the patient, with the reassurance that it is due neither to brain disease nor an indication of impending stroke – anxieties that may have provoked the undesirable emotional response, causing negative feedback that encourages a patient to pay undesirable subconscious attention to the symptom, and which may have been unfortunately enhanced by inappropriate medical advice.

Tinnitus maskers, which look like hearing aids, were used for many years to render the tinnitus inaudible. Now it is realized that continued detection of the tinnitus must be maintained, and indeed that masking is harmful. Patients must avoid silence and experience their symptom in the presence of an emotionally neutral sound background, provided by low-level broad-band sound, for the effective acquisition of the tinnitus habituation that is the aim of treatment. In the majority of patients, this can be achieved within 18 months.

Further reading

Graham J, Martin M. (eds) (2001) *Ballantyne's Deafness, 6th Edition*. Whurr Publishers Ltd, London.

Jastreboff PJ, Hazell JWP. (2004) *Tinnitus Retraining Therapy Implementing the Neurophysiological Model*. Cambridge University Press, Cambridge.

Further resources

British Tinnitis Association website, www. tinnitis.org.uk

CHAPTER 4

Adult Hearing Rehabilitation and Cochlear Implants

Kevin Gibbin

OVERVIEW

Rehabilitation uses:

- Tactics
- Hearing aids
- Environmental aids
- Cochlear impants.

It is estimated that, of the greater than 20 million Britons over the age of 50, 40% have some degree of hearing loss. Not all hearing loss equates to disability, but nonetheless it is clear that there is a large ageing population increasingly likely to need hearing support. That support may be provided in one or more of a number of ways depending on individual need. A small number of those with adult-onset hearing loss may be helped surgically, for example those with otosclerosis and some with chronic infective middle ear disease.

Hearing tactics

Counselling is an essential part of the management of hearing disability with recognition of the individual patient's circumstances. The following simple elements of advice should be incorporated into the consultation with any patient with a hearing loss.

- Reporting. The listener should make those with whom he/she comes into contact aware of the hearing loss: 'Please speak clearly, I have some difficulty with my hearing'. This will hopefully result in the talker speaking clearly and the listener hearing well, but there is an additional psychological element – if the patient does not catch what is said, then the onus is on the speaker to speak more clearly.
- Positioning. Ideally, the speaker should always be in a good light and facing the patient to facilitate acquisition of visual clues.
- Background noise. Wherever possible this should be kept to a minimum; good acoustic conditions with carpets and soft furnishings help with this.
- Listening in groups. Ideally, only one person should speak at a time.

None of the above should cause embarrassment to either the listener or the speaker(s).

Additional support depends on the degree of the hearing loss suffered and may take the form of hearing aid(s), including vibrotactile devices, cochlear implants and, for a small group of the deaf, sign language. Other provision includes the use of environmental aids as well as specialist rehabilitation, such as that available from a hearing therapist or from a centre such as LINK.

Hearing aids

The mainstay of auditory rehabilitation for adults with hearing disability is the use of a hearing aid for one or both ears. A great variety of aids is available both from the private sector and from the National Health Service (NHS). Almost all aids provided through the NHS are behind the ear (BTE) aids, although the facility exists in the NHS to provide in the ear models where appropriate and required for medical reasons, for example in a patient with a deformed pinna who is not able to wear a BTE aid. Many aids issued in the private sector are in the ear models of various types, ranging from tiny devices that are contained within the external auditory canal (in the canal aids) to the slightly larger models that fit within the conchal fossa (in the ear models) (Fig. 4.1). For BTE aids, a range of different types of ear-mould are available and a range of different materials may be used, including non-allergenic ones. In the case of BTE aids, some form of tubing is required in order to conduct the amplified sound to the ear.

Modification of the mould and connecting tubing can be used as a further means of tuning the aid to the patient's audiometric profile. It is a fundamental requirement that the moulds be a good fit, especially for the more high-powered and in the ear aids, to avoid sound 'leaking' around the mould and causing the typical high-pitched squeal of positive acoustic feedback.

Increasingly, the technology in the aid provided is digital, with fewer analogue aids being fitted (Fig. 4.2). The benefit of digital aids is that they are programmable to map to the patient's audiometric hearing loss closely in order to amplify sound more selectively. This is achieved by the incorporation of many channels within the aid, accomplished by the use of selective (band-pass) electronic filters, each capable of independent tuning. The more sophisticated aids available incorporate noise reduction strategies to help boost ease of listening to speech in noisy surroundings.

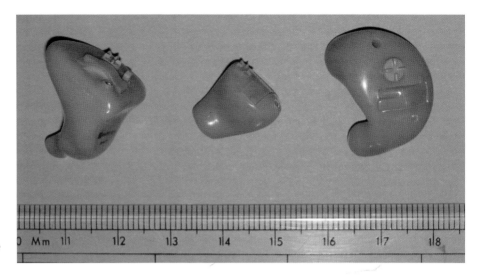

Figure 4.1 In the ear (left and right) and in the canal (centre) hearing aids.

Both digital and analogue aids issued through the NHS (Fig. 4.3) are supplied on contract by all the major manufacturers.

All aids have four discrete components:

- microphone;
- amplifier;
- receiver;
- power supply/battery.

Most aids incorporate the facility to receive radio-frequency signals for reception in public places such as theatres, which may be fitted with a loop system, in effect bypassing acoustic transmission and avoiding much of the background noise otherwise inherent in the surroundings. Use of the T setting on the aid provides this, and the same system may be used for appropriately fitted telephone receivers. Another technology now used in aids is Bluetooth, allowing a wireless link with the growing assortment of Bluetooth signal sources.

Hearing aids are available for a variety of special circumstances. Some patients with a unilateral hearing loss may benefit from a contralateral routing of signal (CROS) fitting, the aid being fitted to the good ear, with the microphone on the opposite side. Of course, for those with a bilateral loss, a binaural fitting may be provided with the potential benefit of including some degree of sound localization and better hearing in noisy surroundings.

Some patients with chronic or incipient ear infections may find wearing an aid in the affected ear difficult, with increased likelihood of discharge. In these cases, a bone-anchored hearing aid (BAHA) may be provided, utilizing the now well-tried technology of osseo-integration achieved by intraosseous titanium implants. A titanium fitting is inserted into the bone adjacent to the pinna, with a surrounding area of non-hair-bearing skin. The BAHA clips onto this via a snap coupling. This technology is also available to those with other conditions, such as bilateral congenital absence of the ear canal. Although still available, vibrotactile aids are used less and less as cochlear implants become more widely available.

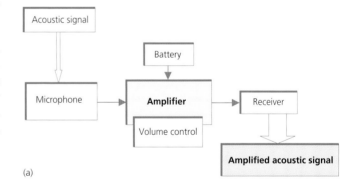

(a)

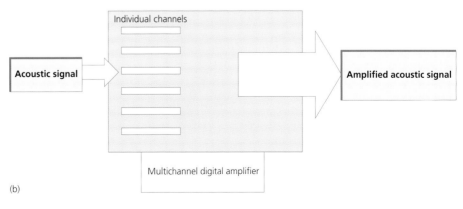

(b)

Figure 4.2 (a) Block diagram of a simple acoustic hearing aid. (b) Block diagram of a multichannel digital hearing aid.

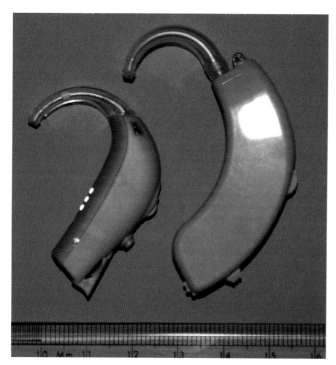

Figure 4.3 NHS hearing aids. Left: digital aid. Right: analogue aid.

Environmental aids

These devices typically provide visual cues or vibration as a surrogate for the auditory signal, for example flashing light door or telephone bells, pagers and smoke alarms. Telephone amplifiers, personal listeners, personal loop systems, infra-red and other television listening devices are available. Textphones (Minilink) telephone message transmission devices can also help the deaf, as can the provision of a hearing dog for the deaf.

Cochlear implants

For those whose hearing loss is so great that they are unable to access audition by acoustic means, a cochlear implant may be appropriate (Fig. 4.4). Cochlear implantation (CI) is predicated on the use of electrical stimulation of the intact acoustic nerve in those cases in which cochlear degeneration has occurred, and relies on the tonoto-

pic organization of the cochlea: that is to say the organization of the cochlea and its nerve supply in a tonal order, high frequencies being detected at the basal end of the cochlea, low frequencies at the apex.

A cochlear implant consists of two major components. The part that is implanted consists of:
- the antenna or aerial, a circular coil;
- the receiver package, which contains electronic circuitry distributing the electrical signal to;
- the electrode array, which is inserted into the cochlea.

The externally worn parts of the cochlear implant comprise:
- a microphone;
- the speech processor that analyses and digitizes the acoustic signal; and
- the transmitter coil, which transmits both the electrical signal and the power for the implanted elements by an FM link. The transmitter coil is co-located with the receiver coil by magnets.

Early cochlear implants were all body worn devices, but now all three major manufacturers provide ear level speech processor systems.

The indication for CI is profound hearing loss demonstrated by the use of both pure tone audiometry and speech recognition tests. The most commonly used such list is the Bamford–Kowal–Bench (BKB) sentence list, and it is now widely accepted that patients who fail to score higher than 40% on this test may prove to be candidates for implantation.

Although there are few contraindications, some considerations are shown below.
- Medical – significant life-limiting disease. CI has been undertaken under local anaesthesia.
- Otological – active ear infection; once treated, patients with such disease may be considered for CI.
- Aetiology of deafness – advanced cochlear obliteration most typically due to meningitis or otosclerosis may present some surgical challenges, but is not an absolute contraindication; special surgical techniques are available for those with cochlear obliteration. Imaging is an important part of the work-up for a CI candidate either with high-resolution CT or MRI in order to demonstrate a hopefully patent cochlear duct.
- Psychological – major psychological or psychiatric disorder. It should however be recognized that deafness itself may engender some psychological problems.

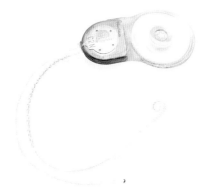

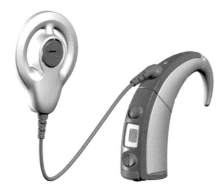

Figure 4.4 Components of a cochlear implant. Left diagram, the implanted components. Right diagram, the externally worn components (courtesy of Cochlear Europe Ltd).

CI surgery has been extensively audited and is safe, although there are risks, and good practice dictates that patients should be warned of these risks shown below.

- Infection – a significant risk as with all implanted foreign bodies; perhaps 0.5%.
- Device failure – relatively high with very early cochlear implants, but now a relatively low risk.
- Facial nerve injury – a very uncommon complication despite surgery in close proximity to the nerves.
- Meningitis – a rare complication, recognized only in the last 2 years; patients are now expected to have received a pneumococcal vaccination as a precaution.

A variety of methods are available to measure the outcome or benefit from CI; these measures may be found in the domain of improvement of communication skills – measured hearing levels, speech perception and production using a number of test batteries; psychological benefit appears to correlate with audiological benefit in many areas assessed. Further benefit may be seen in the area of employment. Cost utility has been assessed and may be compared with coronary artery bypass grafting with a similar cost per QALY (Quality Added Life Year).

Further reading

Cooper H, Craddock L. (2005) *Cochlear Implants: A Practical Guide, 2ⁿᵈ Edition*. Whurr Publishers Ltd, London.

Graham J, Martin M. (eds) (2001) *Ballantyne's Deafness, 6ᵗʰ Edition*. Whurr Publishers Ltd, London.

Further resources

British Cochlear Implant Group, www.bcig.org

British Deaf Association, www.britishdeafassociation.org.uk
   Email: helpline@signcommunity.org.uk

British Society of Audiology, www.thebsa.org.uk
   Email: bsa@thebsa.org.uk

British Society of Hearing Aid Audiologists, www.bshaa.co.uk
   Email: info@bshaa.com

The Hearing Aid Council, www.thehearingaidcouncil.org.uk
   Email: hac@thehearingaidcouncil.org.uk

Hearing Concern, www.hearingconcern.org.uk

International Federation of Hard of Hearing People, www.ifhoh.org

Local and County Councils may also provide information for those with hearing difficulties, for example www.nottinghamshire.gov.uk/socialservices

LINK Centre for Deafened People, www.linkcentre.org
   Email: linkcntr@dircon.co.uk

National Cochlear Implant Users Association, www.nciua.demon.co.uk
   Email: enquiries@nciua.demon.co.uk

Patient UK features a comprehensive range of relevant websites, www.patient.co.uk/showdoc/238

Royal National Institute for Deaf People – for a wide range of environmental aids and other support for deaf adults, www.rnid.org.uk
   Email: solutions@rnid.org.uk

CHAPTER 5

Childhood Hearing Loss

David Albert

OVERVIEW

- Hearing loss in children affects all facets of development, not only speech and language development.
- Significant resources are spent in the Western World for its early detection, diagnosis and rehabilitation. This rehabilitation requires a 'team approach' with good communication between families, community workers and schools.
- Testing for hearing loss must be commenced in the neonate and at any other time when a problem may be suspected.
- Otitis media with effusion (glue ear) is the most common cause of a conductive hearing loss and the majority of cases do not require any surgical interventions. The insertion of a grommet and adenoidectomy are helpful in the immediate short-term resolution.
- Children with a sensorineural hearing loss may be helped by hearing aids or possibly by cochlear implantation.

Introduction

Homo sapiens stands apart with a highly developed system of communication. Any impairment that interferes with our ability to communicate threatens the affected individual's integration into society. Childhood hearing loss is taken seriously by all, and significant resources are expended in prevention, detection and management.

Childhood hearing loss not only affects speech and language development but also cognitive, social and emotional development. The challenge of early detection and intervention in severe and profound sensorineural hearing loss has to be balanced by a more expectant and conservative approach in the commonest type of mild to moderate childhood hearing loss from otitis media with effusion. Technological advances have improved early detection, and paediatric cochlear implantation is nothing short of a miracle. Working with hearing-impaired children requires a team approach and good communication with community workers and schools.

Early detection of hearing loss: universal neonatal screening

Screening only those children with selected risk factors is inefficient, as 95% of children with one or more risk factor(s) will have normal hearing. Conversely, half of children eventually shown to have sensorineural hearing loss will have no risk factors. This realization has

prompted a progressive change to universal neonatal hearing screening. This has been shown to increase detection rates and decrease the age of detection with benefits to speech and language development.

Ideally, screening protocols should only pass neonates with normal hearing, while accepting that some who fail may eventually also be shown to have normal hearing after subsequent testing. The tests should be relatively cheap and require minimal training. Most programmes are based on a mixture of otoacoustic emissions (OAEs) and brain stem evoked responses (BSERs), either using both tests, or a two-tier system with initial screening with OAEs. Support and information must be given to parents whose child has failed a screening test as they wait anxiously for the next-level test.

OAEs are acoustic responses of the cochlea to auditory stimulation. They are present in neonates with normal hearing so long as the external and middle ear are also normal. Middle ear effusions or canal debris can affect the results, as can testing in a noisy environment. OAEs test outer hair cell function, so rare abnormalities of the inner hair cell or auditory nerve will be missed.

BSERs are responses to auditory stimulation recorded from scalp electrodes. The stimulus is a non-frequency-specific click. Automated detection algorithms are used in screening to give a pass/fail equivalent to about 30–35 dB nHL (normal hearing level).

Early provision of hearing aids

Early detection of hearing loss is useless without prompt further assessment, confirmation of loss and, most important, early provision of hearing aids. As well as early aiding, support, information and counselling are needed for the family.

Further investigations in neonatal deafness

Neonates who fail screening, and have a genuine hearing loss confirmed, warrant further investigation. This also includes those who have survived prematurity, as prematurity, without significant hypoxic episodes or ototoxicity, does not itself seem to cause deafness. Investigations should include blood tests as well as an ECG and genetic testing. Protocols are evolving that rely more heavily on genetic testing as this becomes more widely available. Connexin 26 mutations are the commonest cause of non-syndromic deafness, accounting for 50% of all autosomal recessive non-syndromic hearing loss in Caucasians.

Childhood audiometry

Despite universal neonatal hearing screening, it is important to test the hearing of children at older ages as well. This will pick up those who have progressive or acquired sensorineural deafness as well as the common condition of glue ear. Some children will be identified at screening, while others will present to the general practitioner with a suspected hearing loss.

Children from 6 to 18 months can be tested by distraction testing. Here, they sit on their mother's knee with their attention on a visual stimulus in front of them. This stimulus is withdrawn leaving them in a state optimized to receive an auditory stimulus from the side that prompts a head turning response. Properly conducted with an experienced team in a soundproofed room, this can give accurate frequency-specific information for each ear separately. A development is to reward an appropriate head turn with a visual 'treat' such as a moving toy. This is visually reinforced audiometry (Fig. 5.1).

Older children from 2 to 3 years onward can perform conditioned audiometry. They are taught to respond to sounds by performing a task such as putting men in a boat (Fig. 5.2). Once the game is established, the amplitude is reduced to threshold and different frequencies are tested. In the youngest this may have to be free field, but once

headphones are tolerated each ear can be tested accurately. Older children can respond with a button as in adult testing (Fig. 5.3). In the clinic environment, such as in a hospital setting, one would use the digital audiometer (Fig. 5.4) which can give a reliable and objective measure of the hearing in each ear in decibels (dBA).

Impedance testing (with tympanometry) is often used in general practice and school as it is quick and objective, but it does not test hearing. It tests the ability of the middle ear to absorb sound at different ear canal pressures. It can show the presence of middle ear effusions as well as perforated or hypermobile tympanic membranes (Figs 5.5 and 5.6).

Otitis media with effusion/middle ear effusion – 'glue ear'

Middle ear effusions are common in children and may be asymptomatic. Effusions can, however, be associated with frequent recurrent ear infections and/or with significant hearing loss with subsequent

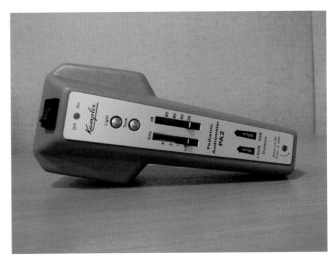

Figure 5.3 Response audiometry – 'button response'.

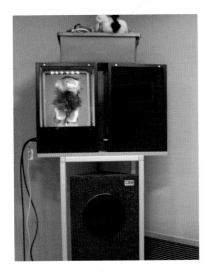

Figure 5.1 Visual enforced audiometer.

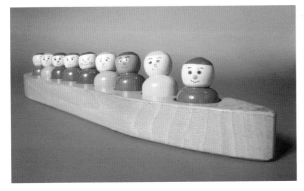

Figure 5.2 Conditioned audiometry – 'putting men in the boat'.

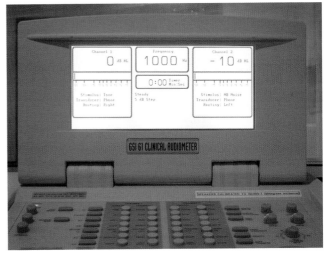

Figure 5.4 Digital audiometry.

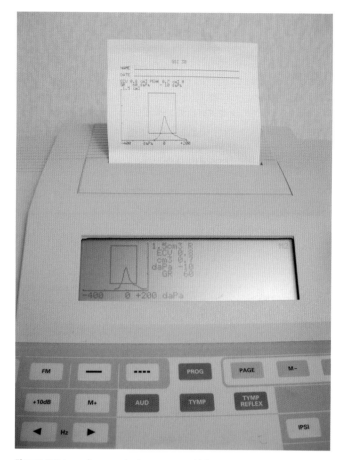

Figure 5.5 Impedence meter to measure middle ear pressures.

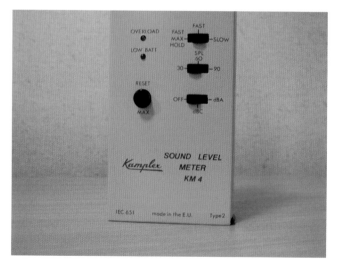

Figure 5.6 Sound pressure meter.

The history is important to assess the impact of the condition in the individual child. A typical presentation with hearing loss would include inattention, variable response to commands, high volume levels for television and poor articulation. The level of competing noise at school or in the home is important as it affects a child's ability to cope with a hearing loss. Speech delay is assessed in young children by vocabulary, articulation and the development of language, as shown by the number of two- to three-word utterances. In older children, articulation is the key area affected by hearing loss in glue ear. Frustration is a common finding in younger children with speech delay secondary to glue ear, with consequent poor behaviour at nursery.

In children with ear infections associated with glue ear, the age of the first infection is a good prognostic indicator of future troubles. It is important to try to decide whether the ears return to normal in between infections – 'discrete infections', whether the infection recurs after a short course of antibiotics – 'inadequately treated infections', or whether separate infections are occurring on a background of quiescent glue ear – 'recurrent infections'. A history of snoring and mouth breathing may suggest associated adenoid hypertrophy.

Examination of the ear may show a dull grey, plum or yellow tympanic membrane (Figs 5.7, 5.8 and 5.9). Fluid levels and bubbles show that at least some air is present in the middle ear. Balance and gait may be affected. Simple conversational tests in the office are a useful guide to help parents to understand the level of hearing loss from glue ear.

Age-appropriate audiometry is important, although levels will fluctuate as glue ear is a seasonally fluctuating condition. The pattern seen on tympanometry affects the likelihood of an effusion being present. The flat line 'B' type trace has an 80% likelihood of effusion, whilst the 'normal' 'A' trace has less than 5% chance of an effusion.

Treatment is expectant, medical or surgical. A period of 3 months of 'watchful waiting' is recommended. If presentation is delayed, this period may have elapsed by the time of presentation. During

speech, language, social and educational delay. It is clear that 'glue ear' is not a discrete condition with a simple management plan that fits all. As it is common and self-limiting, the initial approach to investigation and intervention should be conservative and should generally include a period of 'watchful waiting'. Glue ear is age-related and coincides with the incidence of seasonal upper respiratory tract infections.

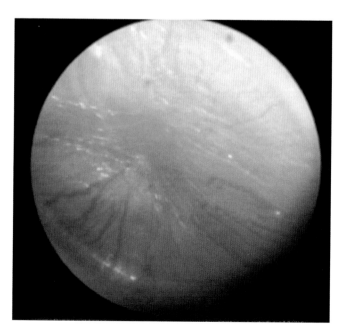

Figure 5.7 Normal tympanic membrane.

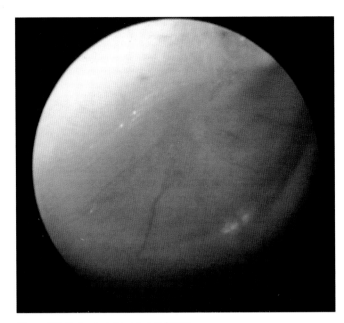

Figure 5.8 Dull grey tympanic membrane.

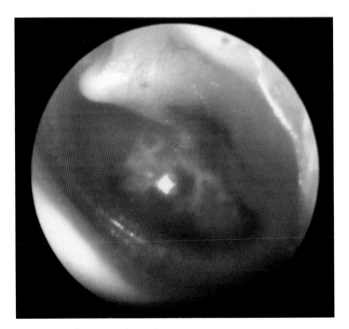

Figure 5.9 Yellow tympanic membrane.

the waiting period, cow-protein-free diets can be tried, particularly in younger children with a history of atopy. There is no evidence to support cranial osteopathy for glue ear. Medical treatment with antibiotics or steroids has not been shown to effect long-term cure. Long courses of low-dose broad-spectrum antibiotics (such as Co-Amoxiclav) have a small, medium-length benefit in clearing effusions, but are particularly useful in controlling the infections in recurrent acute otitis media with effusion. There may also be some benefit from nasally inhaled steroids in those with coexistent allergy. Medically, it would seem reasonable to offer antibiotics if glue ear is associated with infections.

Tympanostomy tubes (grommets)

Surgical drainage of middle ear effusions alone gives a short-lived benefit with reaccumulation of fluid in most cases within six weeks. Laser myringotomy under local anaesthesia is not practical in most children. Surgical treatment for most children consists of drainage followed by placement of a ventilation tube (Fig. 5.10), which typically will stay in place for up to a year. After this time, there is little long-term benefit of ventilation tubes, unless tubes that are designed to stay longer are used. These typically have a higher chance of being complicated by a perforation.

Many protocols have been developed to decide which children with glue ear should be offered tubes. A moderate hearing loss of over 30 dB is a fair consensus, but the effect of the loss on the child and, in particular, on speech delay is a factor. Educational difficulties and behavioural problems from frustration with poor speech all need to be considered in a balanced decision with parental guidance. Parents should be offered alternatives i23 cluding no treatment or amplification. They need to realize that the tubes are designed to be extruded and that a proportion of children may need a further set of tubes.

The majority of children suffer few complications from tube insertion other than occasional discharge and perforation, and minor tympanosclerosis of the membrane, which does not usually affect the hearing. Major anaesthetic complications in children undergoing tube insertion alone have not been reported.

Discharge should be sent for culture and, if the discharge persists, a short course of antibiotic ear drops needs to be used. Some are ototoxic, although it is uncertain whether this is a theoretical or genuine but very rare risk. Topical ciprofloxacin available as eye drops is safe and effective for *Pseudomonas*.

There is no clear evidence of any risk that should stop children swimming, which is an important life skill and part of school life for

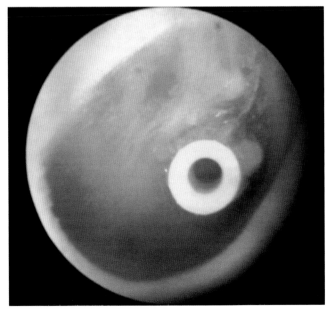

Figure 5.10 Grommet *in-situ*, right tympanic membrane.

many. A few children have repeated episodes of discharge and this group should probably wear silicone or customized ear plugs, drying the canal after swimming with a hair dryer if practical.

Children with tubes need a follow-up to check normalization of the audiogram, and further checks until the tube has been extruded to identify rare sequelae such as cholesteatoma and perforation.

Adenoidectomy

Adenoidectomy helps resolution of glue ear, even if the adenoids are not enlarged and there are no symptoms of obstruction. Combining adenoidectomy with tube insertion offers the medium-term benefit of ventilation tubes with the longer-term benefit of adenoidectomy. Newer techniques, such as suction diathermy, avoid bleeding and have a very low recurrence rate. There remains the small risk of hypernasality, which may be an expression of a submucous cleft palate.

Other causes of conductive deafness in children

Conductive deafness in the absence of perforation or effusion is due to ossicular fixation or discontinuity. Both are rare in non-syndromic children. Children, such as those with Treacher-Collins, Apert's, Crouzon's, CHARGE, Down's or hemifacial microsomia, can be affected. In some, the outer ear and pinna are unaffected, but in others there is a variable degree of canal stenosis or atresia and microtia.

Bone-anchored hearing aids for conductive hearing loss

These aids stimulate the intact cochlea by bone conduction, bypassing any cause of conductive deafness and avoiding the problems of bone-conducting aids of the 'Alice band' type. They are used when a conventional aid cannot be employed because of meatal atresia or discharge. Originally developed for dental implants, osseointegration techniques allow secure fixation of hearing aids with a fixture surrounded by living bone and no intervening capsule. They penetrate the skin without infection. The aids are mounted on the fixture with a quick-release collar or abutment. Placing the fixture usually requires one or two procedures and the site needs to be kept clean. The hearing benefit is excellent.

Cochlear implants for profound hearing loss

In some children, hearing loss is so severe that they derive little benefit from conventional hearing aids (See Chapter 4). This group can be helped by direct stimulation of the auditory nerve with a multichannel implanted wire within the cochlea. Sound is picked up externally by a microphone and amplified, filtered and coded in the external speech processor. The coded signal is then relayed to an implanted device by an external coil held in place with a magnet.

The internal device deciphers the coded signal and separates it into the different channels of the wire within the cochlea. The signal is based on speech, but is not just an amplified and filtered speech signal. Different strategies have been developed to code the signal that is presented to the channels of the implant, which represent regions of the cochlea. Even adults who lose hearing but already have speech take time to interpret the coded signal. Children implanted very early, before they have developed speech, tend to do very well because of the tremendous plasticity of the brain at that early stage. At present, the lower age of implantation in congenital deafness is about a year. Below this it is difficult to establish hearing levels and to have an effective trial of hearing aids. In a situation that mirrors the gradual provision of bilateral hearing aids, the provision of bilateral cochlear implants is becoming more common. As the technology improves, and surgery becomes ever more routine, the level of hearing loss that justifies a cochlear implant is gradually decreasing, so that now children are implanted who *could* gain benefit from conventional aids but who will gain *more* benefit from an implant.

Education and support

Any child with a persistent hearing loss will benefit from experienced, professional support in the educational environment to ensure that teachers are aware of the extent of the loss and how best to overcome it. FM signals from a teacher's microphone received by the child's hearing aid give clear sound without the amplified background noise that bedevils conventional hearing aid use.

The future is very bright for hearing-impaired children, with technology constantly improving conventional aids and cochlear implants. In time it may be possible to regenerate lost hair cells to improve hearing in a truly remarkable and physiological way.

Further reading

Lous J, Burton M, Fielding JU, Ovesen T *et al.* (2005) Grommets (ventilation tubes) for hearing loss associated with otitis media with effusion in children. *Cochran Database Syst Rev*; **25**(1): CD001801 Review.

Maw R, Bawden R. (1993) Spontaneous resolution of severe chronic glue ear in children and the effect of adenoidectomy, tonsillectomy, and the insertion of ventilation tubes (grommets) *Br Med J*; **306** (6880): 756–60.

Medical research council multicentric otitis media study group. (2001) Surgery for persistent otitismedia with effusion: generalizability of results from the UK trial (TARGET). trial of alternative regimens in glue ear treatment. *Clin Otolaryngol Allied Sci*; **26** (5): 417–24.

Rovers MM, Black N, Browning GG *et al.* (2005) Grommets in otitis media with effusion: an individual patient data analysis. *Arch Dis Child*; **90**(5): 480–5 Review.

Uus K, Bamford J. (2006) Effectiveness of population-based newborn hearing screening in England. Ages of interventions and profile of cases. *Paediatrics*; **117** (5): e887–93.

Wilks J, Maw R, Peters TJ, Harvey I, Golding J. (2000) Randomised controlled trial of early surgery versus watchful waiting for glue ear: the effect on behavioural problems in pre-school children. *Clin Otolaryngol Allied Sci*; 25 (3): 209–14.

CHAPTER 6

Acoustic Neuromas and other Cerebello Pontine Angle Tumours

Anthony Wright

OVERVIEW

- Acoustic schwanomas (neuromas) to be considered in any patient with unilateral sensorineural symptoms. Some grow to kill by brain stem compression and raised intracranial pressure
- Rarely a feature of neurofibromatosis
- Other tumours include meningiomas

The cerebello pontine angle

The cerebello pontine angle (CPA) is a tapered space between the side wall of the base of the skull and the brain stem and cerebellum. The roof is the tentorium, the tough membrane that separates the posterior cranial fossa from the middle cranial fossa. The CPA is filled with cerebrospinal fluid (CSF) and has sensory and motor nerves crossing it on their way to and from the brain (see Table 6.1 and Fig. 6.1). A major branch of the basilar artery, the anterior inferior cerebellar artery (AICA), courses through the CPA and itself has branches to the pons and to the labyrinth. It ends up supplying the cerebellum in part.

The acoustic and vestibular nerve bundle runs across the middle of the CPA from the inner ear to the brain stem. It arises from the sensory epithelium of the cochlea and vestibular labyrinth. There is one acoustic nerve bundle but three vestibular nerve branches, superior, inferior and singular, which join and then fuse with the acoustic nerve close to the brain stem. The facial nerve runs out from the brain stem a little ahead of the acoustic and vestibular, but all the nerves run through the internal auditory meatus or canal (IAM or IAC) in the petrous temporal bone (Figs 6.2 and 6.3). The facial nerve takes a complex path through the bone turning first forwards at the geniculate ganglion, then backwards across the middle ear, then downwards through the mastoid bone and finally forwards again through the parotid gland on its way to the muscles of facial expression (see Chapter 8).

Table 6.1 Simple description of the nerves of the cerebello pontine angle and their major functions

Cranial nerve	Name	Motor effects	Sensory supply	Special features
IV	Trochlear	Superior oblique moves eye down and medially		Failure causes double vision on looking down and inwards
VI	Abducent	Lateral rectus moves eye to side		Failure causes double vision on side gaze
V	Trigeminal	Chewing	Facial and scalp skin	Initial irritation causes atypical trigeminal neuralgia
VII	Facial	Facial expression	Taste: anterior tongue	Tear glands, salivary glands
VIII	Acoustic		Hearing	
VIII	Vestibular		Balance	
IX	Glossopharnygeal	Palate, swallowing	Taste: back of tongue/palate	Severe difficulty in swallowing and speaking with inhalation because of an incompetent larynx
X	Vagus	Swallowing and speech	Palate, throat	With above
XI	Accessory	Sternomastoid and trapezius muscles		In paralysis the shoulder drops and the arm cannot be lifted properly
XII	Hypoglossal	Motor supply to the same side of the tongue		In paralysis the tongue deviates to the same side

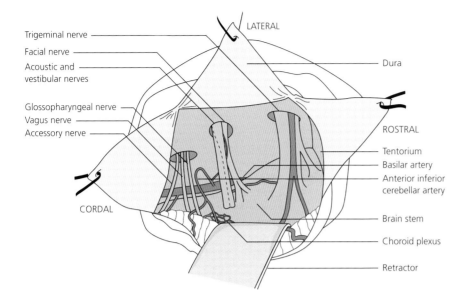

Figure 6.1 Diagram of left cerebello pontine angle and its contents.

Growths in the CPA

With the diversity of structures in the CPA, it is not surprising that many different tumours can grow there. Fortunately, most of them are benign and by far the most common is the doubly misnamed acoustic neuroma. Not only do these usually develop on the superior vestibular nerve, but also they are tumours of the nerve sheath cells – the Schwann cells – which make the myelin sheets that insulate the nerve fibres. Thus they should correctly be called vestibular schwannomas, and any web search should include this term or the term neurilemmomas, which is also sometimes used by purists and pedants. They seem to arise from a single defect on the long arm of chromosome 22, and rarely, if ever, become malignant, although with continued growth they can cause death by brain stem compression.

The incidence of acoustic neuromas has usually been quoted as 1 in 100 000 per year. With improved imaging and greater awareness of the condition, the incidence seems to be increasing slightly. However, the postmortem prevalence is still much higher, which suggests that many people go to their graves with these tumours rather than because of them (see below under diagnosis).

The next most common growth is a meningioma, which arises from the meninges of the inner surface of the skull in this region.

They are generally slow growing and of low-grade malignancy. The other lesions that can occasionally be found in the CPA are listed in Table 6.2.

A particularly unpleasant manifestation of the acoustic neuroma is as a part of the syndrome called neurofibromatosis type 2 (NF2). This is an autosomal dominant condition, classically presenting in youth, with bilateral acoustic neuromas, other neuromas (especially spinal), meningiomas and even gliomas. Fortunately, this condition is rare with an estimated annual incidence of 1 in 2 355 000.

The natural history of acoustic neuromas

Some years ago, it was thought that all acoustic neuromas grew relentlessly so that small tumours eventually became large tumours, which would in turn start to compress the brain stem and cause clumsiness (ataxia) due to cerebellar malfunction. As the brain stem was further compressed, CSF circulation was compromised, and raised intracranial pressure (RICP) developed (see below for symptoms) before inevitable death. This process explained the need for surgical intervention in nearly all cases, despite the risks.

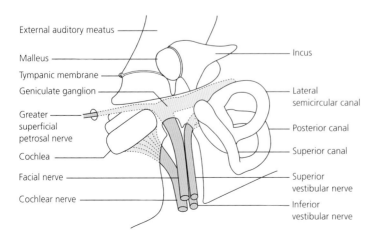

Figure 6.2 Diagram of the right petrous bone and the internal auditory meatus as seen from above.

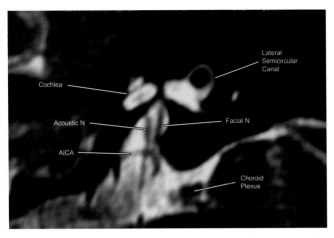

Figure 6.3 Axial MRI scan of normal cerebello pontine angle. AICA, anterior inferior cerebellar artery; N, nerve.

Table 6.2 Lesions in the cerebello pontine angle and their frequency of occurrence

Type	Percentage
Acoustic neuromas	75 minimum
Meningiomas	6
Cholesteatomas	6
Gliomas	3
Others (metastatic tumours, osteomas, osteogenic sarcomas, neuromas of V, VII or IX, angiomas, papillomas of choroid plexus, teratomas, lipomas)	10 maximum

However, it has become clear from long-term observational studies of acoustic neuromas that perhaps 50% or more do not grow over a 10-year period. Like many benign lesions, acoustic neuromas have a 'life span'. They grow at an erratic and very variable rate and eventually stop growing. The irregular growth may be because of a poor blood supply in the surrounding CSF or other intrinsic factors. Some tumours seem to continue to grow relentlessly and cause progressive symptoms, whereas others seem never to grow after diagnosis. It has recently been found that, if small intracanalicular neuromas, i.e. in the internal auditory canal, do not grow over five years, then they do not grow over a subsequent 20-year period. Unfortunately, there do not at present seem to be any clues as to which neuromas will grow and which have finished growing. Of those that do grow, the rate is variable, but quoted figures are often in the range of 1–2 mm in diameter per year.

The symptoms and signs of acoustic neuromas

Many individuals with acoustic neuromas may not have any symptoms at all. Of those that do present to doctors, there seem to be two groups – those that present with relatively minor otological symptoms and those that present with major neurological problems secondary to brain stem compression or the involvement of the trigeminal nerve (V) or the lower cranial nerves (IX, X, XI).

The symptoms that cause referral to an ENT surgeon are outlined in Table 6.3, and to a neurologist or neurosurgeon in Table 6.4 and Box 6.1. The duration of the symptoms has no relationship to the

size of the tumour. The important thing to do is to take unilateral symptoms seriously and investigate them.

Any patient with unilateral sensorineural symptoms must be considered as possibly having an acoustic neuroma.

Diagnosis

Diagnosis relies on the history and examination with appropriate investigations. An ENT examination and pure tone audiogram, along with an examination of the cranial nerves and cerebellar function, will often suggest the possibility of a CPA mass. The next examination is an MRI scan. A T2-weighted fast spin echo (T2FSE) or turbo spin echo (T2TSE) protocol can be used to exclude or confirm a tumour, whilst a gadolinium-enhanced T1 sequence will give more

Table 6.3 Typical presenting symptoms of a patient with an acoustic neuroma sent to ENT Surgeons

Symptom	Primary complaint *	Secondary complaint *
Unilateral alterations in hearing (distortion, hearing loss, tinnitus)	60	16
Headache	16	15
Unsteadiness	7	30
Unilateral fifth nerve symptoms	7	15
Unilateral earache	4	4
Vertigo	3	3
Unilateral sudden profound hearing loss	2	1

* Percentage of patients with acoustic neuromas who cite these symptoms as their primary or secondary complaints
The symptoms that may result in referral to a neurologist are shown in Table 6.4, and are the result of compression of nearby structures

Table 6.4 Symptoms that can arise from compression of nearby structures

Symptom	Structure
Atypical trigeminal neuralgia	V
Tic douloureux	V
Progressive painless facial weakness	VII
Hearing loss and tinnitus on non-tumour side	Brain stem
Hoarse weak voice/dysphagia	X

If the tumour is large enough to block the flow of cerebrospinal fluid (CSF) then the generalized features of raised intracranial pressure (RICP) from an expanding space-occupying lesion in the skull become apparent and referral to a neurosurgeon frequently occurs. The features are shown in Box 6.1

Box 6.1 **Symptoms arising from raised intracranial pressure**

Progressive symptoms are:
- clumsiness, poor balance
- headache
- vertigo
- vomiting
- fevers
- deterioration in mental state
- visual changes
- fits.

information about the nature of the lesion. Figures 6.4 and 6.5 show typical findings.

Management

Large tumours with brain stem compression and incipient RICP

There is little disagreement about these patients who need reduction of the intracranial pressure with some form of shunt and then removal or subtotal removal of the tumour (Fig. 6.6). Whether there should be total removal or subtotal depends on the factors outlined in the following section.

Small- and medium-sized tumours without major neurological symptoms

Given that many tumours do not grow at all and that, even if they do grow, the rate of growth is slow, many consensus groups suggest that the scans should be repeated after 1 year, and, only if there has been growth, should treatment be suggested. This requires proper discussion with the patient and relatives so that an informed decision can be made.

There are three main forms of management, outlined below.

Watch and wait

In the elderly with small, slowly growing tumours, the life expectancy

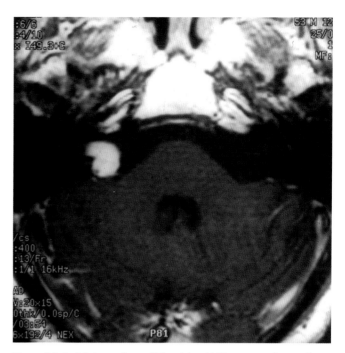

Figure 6.5 Gadolinium-enhanced T1-weighted MRI scan revealing small- to medium-sized acoustic neuroma.

may be shorter than the time that it would take for the tumour to cause threatening neurological problems. A continued programme of monitoring by repeat MRI scans is sometimes recommended.

Stereotactic radiotherapy

Radiation kills tissues, but a single beam directed at an acoustic neuroma is likely to kill everything in its path. Projecting multiple small beams of radiation from different directions that are focused on the tumour reduces the damage to surrounding tissues whilst maximizing the dose in the tumour. This is called stereotactic radiotherapy (SRT). The total dose to be given is calculated from the tumour volume and then given in divided doses over 3 or 4 weeks. This is fractionated SRT. Alternatively, the dose can be given in a single session. As gamma rays are usually used for this protocol, the procedure is misleadingly called gamma knife treatment and the technique

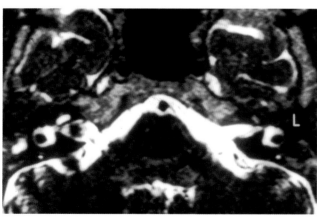

(a)

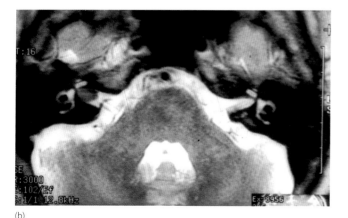

(b)

Figure 6.4 Two axial MRI scans showing small intracanalicular acoustic neuromas of the right internal auditory meatus. T2-weighted scan.

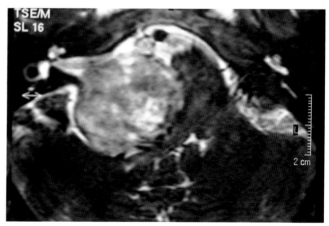

Figure 6.6 T2-weighted spin echo MRI showing large right acoustic neuroma with significant brain stem compression.

radiosurgery. This is misleading, because the tumour is not removed – rather, its growth is slowed or stopped.

The risks of SRT are:

- it fails to work and the tumour continues to grow, after which surgery is extremely difficult because of scarring;
- there is radiation-induced damage to nearby structures – especially the facial nerve and brain stem;
- a long-term risk of malignant change, which may make it unadvisable in the young.

Despite these reservations and lack of tissue diagnosis, SRT is a valuable form of treatment, and is being used increasingly.

Surgery

The aim of surgery is complete removal of the tumour, with no added neurological deficit. Unfortunately, this is difficult to achieve with larger tumours and even with small ones there is risk. Damage to the facial nerve, which is stretched around the capsule of the tumour, is the main risk. Even if the dissection is meticulous and the nerve is anatomically intact, it sometimes fails to function. A facial paralysis is particularly distressing and anything more than minor damage (House–Brackmann grade III or more – see Chapter 8) causes a major reduction in the quality of life. The risk of a facial paralysis increases with the size of the tumour. To reduce this risk, many surgeons now undertake a subtotal removal of the tumour, leaving a strip of capsule on the nerve to protect it. The patient then has serial scans to detect if there is growth of the remnant. If there is, further surgery or radiotherapy could be contemplated when the mass reaches a significant size (Figs 6.7 and 6.8).

The surgical approaches are outlined below.

- Transmastoid/translabyrinthine. The IAM and CPA are approached through the mastoid and, in turn, by removing the bony inner ear. This minimizes traction on the brain, but hearing is lost.
- Retrosigmoid/suboccipital. The craniotomy is made behind the sigmoid sinus with the cerebellum retracted for access. The surgical view is shown in Fig. 6.1. With small tumours less than 1.5 cm, it may be possible to preserve hearing. The IAC has to be opened by drilling to remove tumour within it
- Middle cranial fossa approach. The craniotomy is made above the ear into the middle fossa, and small intracanalicular tumours can

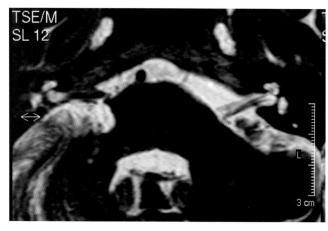

Figure 6.8 Same patient as in Fig. 6.7, 1 year following operation. There is a small area of residual neuroma/capsule on the VIIth nerve. Notice how the fourth ventricle has returned to a normal shape.

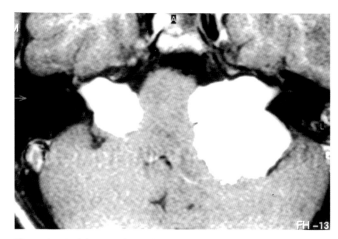

Figure 6.9 Gadolinium-enhanced MRI scan showing bilateral acoustic neuromas. Material on the right has been partly removed (elsewhere).

be removed with preservation of hearing. The temporal lobe has to be retracted for access. This approach is used less in Europe (although several centres in Europe carry out middle fossa surgery) because of the risks of epilepsy – in the UK patients must not drive for a year after such a procedure.

Neurofibromatosis type 2

The management of this difficult condition needs a team approach with ENT surgeons and neurosurgeons working with hearing therapists, genetic counsellors and a social support network to deal with the problems as they arise. The MRI scan in Fig. 6.9 shows large bilateral acoustic neuromas. The tumour on the right side had been partly decompressed, but there is now clear brain stem compression and the risk of hydrocephalus.

Further reading

British Association of Otorhinolaryngologists, 2001. Acoustic Neuromas, Clinical Effectiveness Guidelines: www.entuk.org/publications

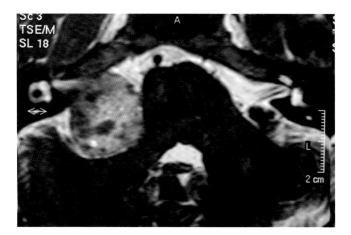

Figure 6.7 Large right-sided acoustic neuroma with some distortion of the fourth ventricle and displacement of the brain stem. Pre-operative scan.

CHAPTER 7

Vertigo

Harold Ludman

OVERVIEW

Vertigo is the symptom of vestibular disturbance and is caused by:

- intrinsic labyrinthine diseases – Menière's disease, benign paroxysmal positional vertigo and acute vestibular failure;
- spread of disease from infected middle ears to the labyrinth;
- disease of the brain stem or cerebellum;
- general systemic conditions affecting the vestibular system.

Vertigo is an illusion of movement, where the patient, or the environment, seems to be moving. Imbalance always accompanies vertigo, but is not always due to vertigo and is not a synonym for vertigo.

Normal balance requires: (a) accurate sensory information from the eyes, proprioceptive receptors and the vestibular labyrinth; (b) coordination of this information within the brain; and (c) a normal motor output from the central nervous system to an intact musculoskeletal system (Fig. 7.1). A fault in any of these impairs balance.

Vertigo arises if information from vestibular sources conflicts with that from the other sensory systems, or when a disordered central integration system in the brain does not correctly assess the body's movements from vestibular input. Vertigo is always a symptom of vestibular defect. This may lie in the peripheral labyrinth or in its connections within the brain. When severe it is accompanied by nausea and vomiting.

Vertigo is caused by: (a) peripheral vestibular disorders (labyrinthine); (b) spread to the labyrinth of infection from middle ear disease; (c) central vestibular disorders, such as multiple sclerosis, tumours, infarcts; and (d) external insults to the vestibular system by drugs, anaemia, hypoglycaemia, hypotension, viral infection (Box 7.1).

The commonest peripheral vestibular disorders are Menière's disease and other forms of endolymphatic hydrops, benign paroxysmal positional vertigo, sudden vestibular failure and vascular disturbances (Box 7.2).

Menière's disease

This is a disorder of endolymph control associated with dilatation of the endolymphatic spaces of the membranous labyrinth (Fig. 7.2). Dilatation, or endolymphatic hydrops, may be caused by disorders of the otic capsule, but in Menière's disease it is, by definition, idiopathic.

The disease usually affects only one ear, first producing symptoms between the ages of 30 and 60. It is characterized by attacks of violent paroxysmal vertigo, often rotatory, associated with deafness and

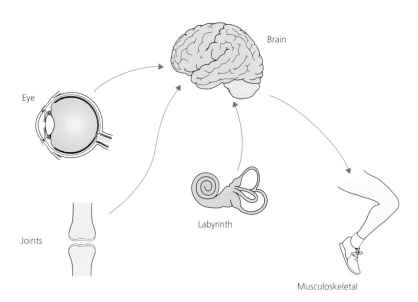

Eye

Brain

Joints

Labyrinth

Musculoskeletal

Figure 7.1 Sensory and motor components of balance.

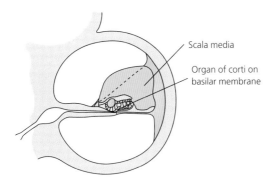

Figure 7.2 Menière's disease – dilated scala media in cochlea.

tinnitus. Attacks occur in clusters with periods of remission, during which balance is normal. Each lasts for several hours, rarely less than 10 minutes or more than 12 hours (Box 7.3), and is accompanied by prostration, nausea and vomiting. A sensation of pressure in the ear, increase or change in the character of tinnitus, pain in the neck or increased deafness often precedes an attack.

The accompanying deafness is sensorineural and fluctuates noticeably in severity. It is associated with distortion of speech and musical sounds, and with severe discomfort on exposure to loud noise (hyperacusis). The hearing loss may precede the first attack, although both symptoms arise together. The vertigo may be so consuming that the hearing loss is not noticed. Hearing improves during remission, but gradually deteriorates, until its impairment becomes severe. The tinnitus is roaring, low pitched and worse when hearing is most impaired.

In at least 20–30% of patients, disease is bilateral and deafness tends to become more serious than the vertigo. A form known as vestibular hydrops produces attacks of episodic vertigo without auditory symptoms. Another variant of Menière's disease is cochlear hydrops, which is a very common cause of fluctuating hearing loss, with tinnitus and distortion, but without vertigo.

Treatment of Menière's disease

Medical treatment with vasodilatory drugs such as betahistine may be useful. Nicotinic acid in a dose sufficient to cause flushing is an alternative. Menière's disease might be associated with electrolyte imbalance, and so a salt-restricted diet combined with a diuretic is often recommended.

Operation is advised if the symptoms are not controlled by medication. Conservative surgical procedures aim to protect hearing, and include decompression of the endolymphatic sac and selective division of the vestibular branch of the vestibulocochlear nerve (vestibular neurectomy). Labyrinthectomy, with total destruction of the membranous labyrinth, guarantees relief from the vertigo but at the expense of total loss of hearing in that ear. This is often acceptable if the hearing remains only as a painful distorted shred in the affected ear when the other is normal.

Benign paroxysmal positional vertigo

Benign paroxysmal positional vertigo (BPPV) is the commonest cause of vertigo (Box 7.4). It is provoked by movements of the head (Fig. 7.3), usually to one side when turning in bed or on looking upwards. Each attack is violent yet lasts for only a few seconds, and only occurs on assuming the provoking position of the head. There are no auditory symptoms. Episodes usually abate and disappear within a few weeks or months, but they often recur.

This disorder is caused by detachment of otoconia (calcium carbonate crystals) from the otolith organ of the utricle. They fall into the posterior semicircular canal and distort its cupula on provoking head positioning. Both labyrinths may be affected. Causes may be head injury, viral infection or degenerative changes with ageing, but often there is no identifiable explanation.

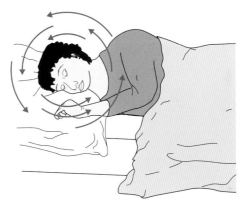

Figure 7.3 Benign paroxysmal positional vertigo.

Treatment of benign paroxysmal positional vertigo

Most patients need no more than reassurance, and avoidance of the provoking head position until recovery. Medication has no useful place. So called 'repositioning' manoeuvres, in which the head is moved through a precise sequence of positions designed to force the displaced otoconia out of the posterior canal into the vestibule, are effective. Some patients are helped by exercises that deliberately provoke the vertigo, to encourage central compensation for the abnormal vestibular stimuli.

Operative measures, only used for rarely persistent severe symptoms, include division of the nerve to the posterior semicircular canal ampulla (singular neurectomy), and obliteration of the lumen of the posterior semicircular canal.

Sudden vestibular failure

Sudden vestibular failure (Fig. 7.4) occurs when one peripheral labyrinth suddenly stops working. This may happen for various reasons – head injuries, viral infection, blockage of an end artery supplying the labyrinth, multiple sclerosis, diabetic neuropathy, or brain stem encephalitis. It is sometimes confusingly referred to as vestibular neuronitis, or epidemic labyrinthitis, terms which are best avoided. The effects are sudden vertigo with prostration, nausea and vomiting. There are no auditory symptoms, and the vertigo persists continuously, gradually improving over many days or weeks. Vertigo is exacerbated by head movements, but after a few days it may be absent unless the head is moved. Patients gradually regain balance so that, on the third or fourth day after onset, they may move unsteadily around the room, holding on to objects for support. By the end of 10 days unsupported walking becomes possible. After 3 weeks gait may seem normal, but patients still feel insecure, particularly in the dark or when tired.

Recovery is slower and less complete in the elderly. It relies on compensating changes within the brain, and imbalance may return temporarily whenever the acquired compensation breaks down – for example, through defects in other sensory systems, fatigue, other illnesses, drugs or the cerebral degeneration of old age.

Migraine

Migraine is a common vascular cause of vertigo and may cause symptoms indistinguishable from vertigo. Basilar migraine, affecting teen-age girls in the main, is also similar, but may be preceded by posterior cerebral arterial symptoms with disturbance of vision, and may be accompanied by dysarthria and tingling in the hands and feet.

Assessment

The first task is to recognize the symptom as vertigo, and then to determine whether there is any systemic cause or extralabyrinthine disorder needing urgent investigation – destructive middle ear disease or any central vestibular abnormalities. The history is especially important.

Clinical examination must include assessment of the cardiovascular and central nervous systems. Careful examination of the ears is the only way to recognize destructive middle ear disease with cholesteatoma. Exclusion demands that each tympanic membrane be found to be normal. A waxy crust over the pars flaccida is deceptive, as it may cork the entrance to an attic cholesteatoma (Fig. 7.5). If in any doubt, referral for examination with a microscope is essential, and anaesthesia may be needed.

Spontaneous jerk nystagmus is always a sign of vestibular disease. Its assessment requires examination of the eyes under good illumination. Inspection in all positions of gaze is necessary, but the eyes should not be abducted more than about 30 degrees – until the edge of the iris reaches the caruncle. Certain characteristics of a jerk nystagmus always indicate a central cause within the brain. These are: (a) nystagmus persisting for more than a few weeks; (b) change in the direction of beat (defined by the direction of quick component) either with time or change in direction of gaze; (c) beating in any direction other than horizontally; (d) different jerks in the two eyes (ataxic).

Stance and gait are examined clinically by watching the patient stand with the eyes closed, and while walking heel to toe.

Positional testing

Simple positional testing is essential as a diagnostic indicator of BPPV. Seated on a couch, the patient turns the head towards the examiner and is told to keep the eyes open, while watching the examiner's forehead. The doctor holds the patient's head, which is rapidly laid back into a supine position with the head over the edge of the

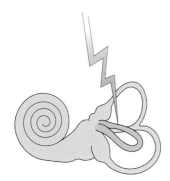

Figure 7.4 Sudden vestibular failure.

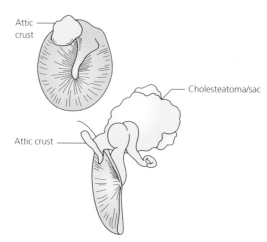

Figure 7.5 Attic crust may obscure cholesteatoma.

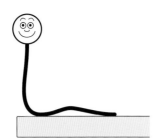

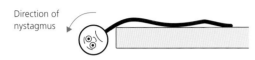

Direction of nystagmus

Figure 7.6 Positional test.

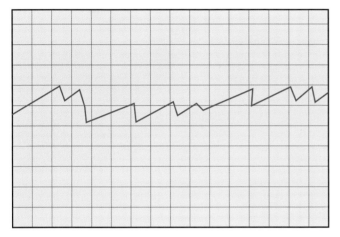

Figure 7.7 Trace of electronystagmography showing left bearing nystagmus.

couch – 30 degrees below horizontal (Fig. 7.6). The patient is held in that position for at least 30 seconds, despite protest, while the patient's eyes should be watched for nystagmus. The test is then repeated with the head turned to the other side. Nystagmus provoked by this is always an abnormal finding.

Positional nystagmus is elicited in BPPV, but it can also, rarely, indicate a vestibular lesion somewhere in the posterior cranial fossa. In BPPV the nystagmus invariably shows the following features: (a) it is rotatory, beating towards the underlying ear; (b) a latent period of some seconds precedes its onset; (c) it abates after 5–20 seconds in the provoking position and is less violent on repeated testing; (d) it is accompanied by violent vertigo; (e) it does not change direction during observation. Deviation from any of these features suggests a central cause, requiring further investigation.

Box 7.5 **Features of central nystagmus**

Central *spontaneous* nystagmus is indicated by:
- persistence for several weeks;
- change in direction (of quick component) with time or direction of gaze;
- direction other than horizontal;
- ataxic beating.

Examination next requires the assessment of hearing (see Chapter 3). Further, more detailed testing entails referral for neuro-otological investigations of vestibular function. These include the caloric test, in which the lateral semicircular canal is vicariously stimulated by irrigation of the ears with water at temperatures other than body temperature, and rotation tests, when the whole body is turned in a specially designed chair at variable angular acceleration. Nystagmus induced by these tests, and also without provocation of any kind, is recorded by electronystagmography (ENG; Fig. 7.7), which proffers valuable diagnostic information about both spontaneous and induced nystagmus (Box 7.5).

Symptomatic treatment of vertigo

Symptoms may be relieved by sedatives such as prochlorperazine, cinnarizine and other antihistamines. Diazepam is also useful. In a severe attack, bedrest will be necessary whatever the cause. Drugs may be given intramuscularly or as suppositories. Once the acute stage is over, sedatives are continued in small doses for several weeks or months.

If vestibular deficit, rather than irritation of a labyrinthine system, is pronounced, vestibular sedatives may exacerbate the symptoms. This often happens in the degenerative changes of old age and in bilateral Menière's disease, or ototoxic damage. Patients can be helped by graded head and eye movement exercises, designed to accelerate the process of central compensation. These head exercises should be taught and supervised by specially trained physiotherapists.

Other treatment is directed at identified causes, including surgical exploration of any middle ear in which cholesteatomatous erosion of the middle ear is suspected.

Further reading

Ludman H, Wright T. (eds) (1998) *Diseases of the Ear, 6th Edition.* Arnold-Hodder Headline, London.

Luxon LM. (ed.) (2003) *Textbook of Audiological Medicine.* Taylor & Francis, London.

CHAPTER 8

Facial Palsy

Iain Swan

OVERVIEW

A lower motor neurone facial palsy is caused by damage to the facial nerve, the VIIth cranial nerve, which supplies the muscles of facial expression.

Anatomy

The facial nerve leaves the facial nucleus in the brain stem and passes through the internal auditory meatus beside the VIIIth cranial nerve. After the geniculate ganglion, it runs across the middle ear in the Fallopian canal and then turns vertically where it supplies the stapedius muscle before leaving the temporal bone through the stylomastoid foramen. It enters the parotid gland where it divides into five main branches to the muscles of facial expression. In the middle ear, it also supplies secretomotor fibres to the submandibular and sublingual salivary glands, and taste fibres to the anterior two-thirds of the tongue via the chorda tympani.

Presentation

Patients present with weakness of the muscles of facial expression (Fig. 8.1). The affected side of the face droops and they may be unable to close their eye. They may complain of hyperacusis due to paralysis of the stapedius muscle. In severe cases, there may be a metallic taste due to loss of taste sensation on one side of the tongue (Fig. 8.2). Reduced lachrymation causes dryness of the affected eye. Poor mouth closure can cause drooling and difficulty with eating.

Most facial palsies are caused by lower motor neurone lesions, but upper motor neurone lesions also occur. In upper motor neurone lesions, the patient can still move the upper part of the face, i.e. the forehead, because of crossover pathways in the brain stem.

Aetiology

Most facial palsies (nearly 75%) are idiopathic. Aetiologies are listed in Table 8.1.

Bell's palsy

Bell's palsy is an idiopathic, lower motor neurone facial palsy. The onset is over a few hours, commonly occurring overnight. Patients

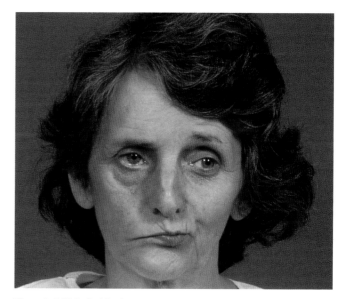

Figure 8.1 Right facial palsy.

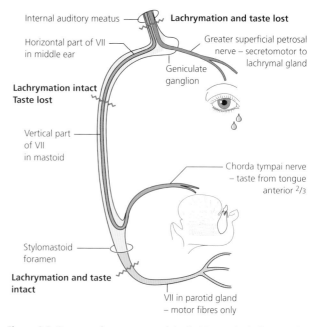

Figure 8.2 Course and components of the facial nerve (VII) - features that help identification of lesion site.

Table 8.1 Aetiologies of facial palsy

Lower motor neurone facial palsy

Idiopathic	Bell's palsy
Infection	Otitis media
	Herpes zoster (Ramsay Hunt syndrome)
	Lyme disease
Neoplasm	Malignant parotid neoplasms
	Middle ear carcinoma
	Facial neuroma
Trauma	
Other	Sarcoidosis
	Multiple sclerosis

Upper motor neurone facial palsy

CVAs
Intracranial tumours

CVA, cerebrovascular incident.

Table 8.2 House–Brackmann grading of facial palsy (House and Brackmann, 1985)

Grade	Definition
I	Normal symmetrical function in all areas
II	Slight weakness noticeable only on close inspection
	Complete eye closure with minimal effort
	Slight asymmetry of smile with maximal effort
	Synkinesis barely noticeable, contracture or spasm absent
III	Obvious weakness, but not disfiguring
	May not be able to lift eyebrow
	Complete eye closure and strong but asymmetrical mouth movement with maximal effort
	Obvious but not disfiguring synkinesis, mass movement or spasm
IV	Obvious disfiguring weakness
	Inability to lift brow
	Incomplete eye closure and asymmetry of mouth with maximal effort
	Severe synkinesis, mass movement, spasm
V	Motion barely perceptible
	Incomplete eye closure, slight movement of corner of mouth
	Synkinesis, contracture and spasm usually absent
VI	No movement, loss of tone, no synkinesis, contracture or spasm

often complain of aching pain around the ear, often preceding the onset of the palsy. Severe otalgia suggests herpes zoster (see below). There may be associated hyperacusis and altered taste. There is an annual incidence of 25–35 cases per 100 000 of the population. Individuals can be affected at any age, but young and middle-aged adults are the most likely to be affected. Pregnant women and individuals with diabetes are thought to be at greater risk.

Aetiology

The symptoms of Bell's palsy arise from inflammation or swelling of the facial nerve. The cause of this in most cases is unknown, although there is some evidence to suggest that some cases are caused by herpes simplex virus (HSV).

Diagnosis

Bell's palsy is a diagnosis of exclusion. The ears and the parotid gland must be carefully examined to exclude middle ear disease and parotid neoplasms. A brief neurological examination will exclude other neurological conditions. The degree of the palsy should be recorded, most commonly using the House–Brackmann grading system (House and Brackmann, 1985; Table 8.2). This is clinically useful as it allows assessment of the patient's progress.

Treatment

The most important part of treatment is advising the patient of the need to protect the affected eye. The eye may become dry, particularly at night, and eye closure may be incomplete. Damage to the cornea may result. Treatment includes artificial tears and an eye patch, or other protective measures, particularly at night and when out of doors on a windy day.

Many doctors prescribe corticosteroids and/or antivirals for Bell's palsies seen within 72 hours of onset. However, Cochrane reviews of steroids (Salinas et al, 2003) and of antivirals (Sipe and Dunn, 2003) have found no good evidence for their efficacy. It is widely agreed that they are of no benefit beyond the first 3–7 days. Hopefully, the question of the efficacy of prednisolone and acyclovir will be answered in 2006 by the Scottish Bell's Palsy Study.

When there is no recovery of facial function, there are surgical procedures to reduce disability. Eye closure can be improved by gold weights in the upper lid and canthal slings. Cross-facial anastomoses can provide innervation to the paralysed facial muscles.

Prognosis

In the majority of cases (70–75%), there is complete recovery of facial function, with partial recovery in a further 10–15% (Adour and Wingerd, 1974). Most patients with Bell's palsy begin to notice improvement in their palsy within 2–3 weeks of the onset of symptoms, although recovery in some patients may be in 3–6 months. The prognosis is better in incomplete palsy (about 95% complete recovery), those with early improvement and younger patients. A small number of cases (3–7%) will have a recurrence of their palsy years later.

If there is no evidence of recovery within 3–4 months, the diagnosis of Bell's palsy should be reconsidered.

Herpes zoster oticus (Ramsay Hunt syndrome)

Ramsay Hunt syndrome is an acute unilateral facial palsy caused by reactivation of varicella zoster virus (VZV) from the geniculate ganglion. It is more common in the immunosuppressed and in the elderly. Patients present with moderate to severe pain around the ear, often with few signs at this stage. They develop a facial palsy, often accompanied by audiovestibular symptoms of hearing loss, tinnitus and vertigo. They usually also have loss of taste on the anterior two-thirds of the tongue. Vesicles usually appear 2–3 days later in the concha (Fig. 8.3) and sometimes on the ipsilateral anterior two-thirds of the tongue and soft palate.

The facial palsy is often more severe than in Bell's palsy. Only 10% of cases with complete facial palsy recover fully if untreated. Early treatment with high-dose antivirals (e.g. acyclovir) and cor-

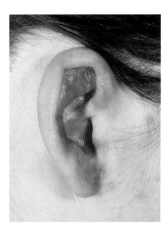

Figure 8.3 Herpes zoster oticus.

ticosteroids (e.g. prednisolone 1 mg/kg per day for 7 days) is important.

Otitis media

Facial palsy is a rare complication of acute suppurative otitis media. Mild weakness can occur in acute otitis media, thought to be due to congenital dehiscence of the facial nerve in the middle ear. This recovers quickly and does not influence the treatment of otitis media.

In chronic suppurative otitis media (CSOM), facial palsy occurs more commonly in active squamous CSOM (cholesteatoma) (Fig. 8.4) but can also occur in mucosal CSOM. It is usually associated with dehiscence of the facial nerve in the Fallopian canal and granulation tissue overlying the nerve. In the presence of a facial nerve palsy, active chronic suppurative otitis media should be managed urgently and almost always surgically. Complete recovery of facial function can be expected in most cases after careful surgical management.

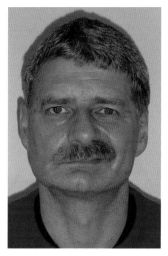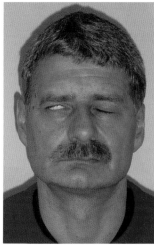

Figure 8.4 Right active squamous chronic otitis media.

Lyme disease

Lyme disease is a rare cause of facial palsy. It is caused by a spirochaete, *Borrelia burgdorferi*, which is transmitted by tick bite in endemic areas of the world. There is a flu-like illness, often with a rash. Cranial neuropathies can occur several weeks later in untreated cases. Facial palsy is the commonest neuropathy and is bilateral in 75% of cases. Treatment is with antibiotics and full recovery is likely.

Neoplasms

Malignant neoplasms of the parotid gland and the middle ear are rare causes of facial palsy. They should be excluded by clinical examination and treated appropriately. Facial neuroma is uncommon. It should be suspected in cases of apparently idiopathic facial palsy which do not recover or continue to progress. It is not a diagnosis which needs to be considered in the early stages of facial palsy, as surgical treatment will usually result in a total facial palsy and, for this reason, is not considered urgent.

Trauma

Facial palsy can occur after head injury with fracture of the temporal bone. Delayed onset palsy, a few hours after injury, is due to swelling around the nerve. Treatment with corticosteroids is recommended and a good recovery is likely. Immediate onset palsy is caused by the nerve being trapped in a fracture line or torn. Surgical exploration should be considered, but the patient's general condition usually precludes this.

Other causes

Facial palsy can occur in sarcoidosis but is a very rare presenting sign. Multiple sclerosis can cause a facial palsy, which can be intermittent; as with other neurological causes, there are usually other signs. Melkerssons syndrome is also another possible cause.

Further reading

Adour KK, Wingerd J. (1974) Idiopathic facial paralysis (Bell's palsy): factors affecting severity and outcome in 446 patients. *Neurology*; **24**: 1112–16.
House JW, Brackmann DE. (1985) Facial nerve grading system. *Otolaryngology – Head & Neck Surgery*; **93**: 146–7.
Murakami S, Mizobuchi M, Nakashiro Y *et al.* (1996) Bell palsy and herpes simplex virus: identification of viral DNA in endoneurial fluid and muscle. *Annals of Internal Medicine*; **124**: 27–30.
Salinas RA, Alvarez G, Alvarez MI, Ferreira J. (2003) Corticosteroids for Bell's palsy (idiopathic facial paralysis). *The Cochrane Database of Systematic Reviews*; **3**.
The Scottish Bell's Palsy Study: Bell's palsy: Early acyclovir and/or prednisolone in Scotland. (BELL'S ISRCTN 71548196). www.dundee.ac.uk/bells/

CHAPTER 9

Paranasal Sinus Diseases and Infections

Parag M Patel, Julian Rowe-Jones

OVERVIEW

- The term rhinosinusitis more accurately describes inflammation of the nose and paranasal sinuses, and terms such a sinusitis and rhinitis should be abandoned.

- Symptoms suggestive of rhinosinusitis are characterised by TWO or MORE of the following symptoms; nasal blockage/congestion, discharge: anterior or postnasal drip, facial pain or pressure and/or a reduction or loss of smell.

- Persistence of symptoms up to 12 weeks are termed acute, and chronic when longer than 12 weeks.

- The causes of rhinosinusitis are many: allergic, infective – viral, bacterial and fungal, as well as non-allergic non-infective, vasomotor, hormonal and drug induced.

- Nasal polyposis is part of the spectrum of chronic rhinosinusitis and is prevalent in 4% of the population, male predominant, increasing with age with peak incidence older than 50 years, with more than 50% having a family history.

- Nasal polyps are typically bilateral – unilateral polyps should be referred to a specialist as they may be a nasal cancer or due to fungal disease.

- Complications of rhinosinusitis though uncommon include periorbital cellulites, intracranial infection – cavernous sinus thrombosis, meningitis, extra and sub dural, as well as frontal lobe abscess, more rare is frontal bone osteomyelitis.

- Treatment should include in the mild to moderate symptomatic patients analgesia, topical decongestants, topical steroids, and only when symptoms are unresolving after 5 days should antibiotics be used.

- In recurrent episodic attacks lasting 7 days or less, consider an allergic cause for symptoms, consider using topical steroids for protracted periods or during the seasonal periods.

- When symptoms are frequent, disabling and not responding to treatments, then consider referring to a specialist. Surgical management may be indicated after investigation or trial of supervised treatment and is currently performed by functional endoscopic sinus surgery (FESS).

- FESS when performed, results in satisfactory relief of symptoms, however recurrences occur and may require further surgery. Complications of such surgery, in the hands of experienced surgeons, are uncommon.

Sinus anatomy and mucociliary pathways

The paranasal sinuses develop in infancy and mature during childhood to pneumatize the midfacial and forehead regions.

At birth, the maxillary sinus is 4–7 mm in diameter. Pneumatization continues at a rate of 2–3 mm/year until full maturity by late adolescence. The maxillary sinus floor is then usually 0.5–1 mm lower than the nasal cavity. There are usually three or four ethmoid sinus cells at birth and these reach their maximum size by age 12. An average adult has 10–15 ethmoid sinus cells.

The sphenoid and frontal sinuses are absent at birth, and develop between 4 and 5 years of age. The sphenoid is fully pneumatized by the age of 8 years, while the frontal sinus reaches maximum volume by age 12 years. There is a group of patients who never develop frontal sinuses.

Within the nasal cavity there are three turbinates: superior, middle and inferior. The air space beneath each turbinate is known as the meatus of the corresponding turbinate. Each group of sinus cells drains into these meatuses: the frontal, maxillary and anterior ethmoid sinuses drain into the middle meatus, the posterior ethmoid sinus drains into the superior meatus, and the sphenoid sinuses drain into the sphenoethmoidal recess at the back of the nasal cavity.

The middle meatus is of special significance as it contains the ostiomeatal complex (OMC). This is an anatomical area in the bony lateral nasal wall comprising narrow, mucosal lined channels and recesses into which the major dependent sinuses drain. The OMC acts physiologically as an antechamber for the frontal, maxillary and anterior ethmoid sinuses. Irritants and antigens are deposited there and may cause mucosal oedema. As the clefts in the OMC are narrow, small degrees of oedema may cause outflow tract obstruction with impaired ventilation of the major sinuses (Figs 9.1 and 9.2).

Nasal epithelium is a pseudostratified columnar ciliated mucous membrane continuous throughout the sinuses. The epithelium contains goblet cells, which produce mucus, and columnar cells with mobile cilia projecting into the mucus, beating 12–15 times a second. The direction of ciliary beats is organized into well-defined pathways, present at birth. These mucociliary pathways ensure drainage of the sinuses through their physiological ostium into the nasal cavity (Fig. 9.3).

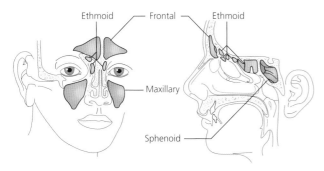

Figure 9.1 Schematic view of the paranasal sinuses.

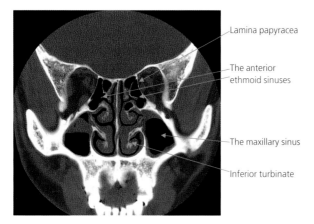

Figure 9.2 Coronal CT scan image of the paranasal sinuses.

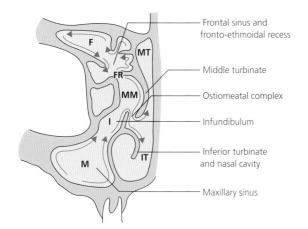

Figure 9.3 Right-sided sinus drainage pathways.

Clinical definition of rhinosinusitis

Nasal and sinus mucosa is continuous and has similar histological features. Patients with rhinitis may well exhibit similar changes in the sinuses and vice versa. The term rhinosinusitis is now more accurately used than rhinitis or sinusitis alone. Disease and associated symptoms may be predominant in either the nose or the sinuses. Rhinosinusitis is defined as inflammation of the nose and the paranasal sinuses characterized by two or more symptoms:

- blockage/congestion;
- discharge: anterior/postnasal drip;
- facial pain/pressure;
- reduction or loss of smell.

Further symptoms may include sneezing, watery rhinorrhoea, nasal and eye itching. Disease up to 12 weeks is termed acute, and chronic thereafter.

Aetiology

Allergy

Allergic rhinosinusitis (AR) may be perennial, seasonal or occupational. Perennial AR is frequently caused by house dust mites (*Dermatophagoides pteronyssinus*); other common causes are cat and dog dander. Seasonal AR may be related to a wide variety of pollens such as grass, tree and weed. Mould spores commonly cause AR. In the spring, oak, elm, birch and grass pollen are most active, whereas in later summer, ragweed and mould spores become a problem. Occupational rhinitis may result from allergy to airborne agents in the workplace, such as latex.

Allergic rhinitis with mucosal oedema in the lateral nasal wall may lead to obstruction of the OMC, reduced ventilation, mucus retention and further pathological changes in the sinus mucosa. This is likely to increase susceptibility to infection.

Pathogenesis of allergy

AR results from IgE-mediated allergy associated with cellular inflammation of the nasal mucosa. Raised levels of eosinophils within the paranasal cavity lead to increased expression of epithelial adhesion molecules, cytokines (IL-4 and IL-5) and chemokines. Resident tissue cells, such as mast cells, release histamine and other mediators.

Infection

Viral

Viral rhinosinusitis (the common cold) has an incubation period of 1–4 days and lasts for up to 7 days. Rhinoviruses and coronavirus are most commonly implicated, but AR can be caused by any type of virus. Primary viral rhinitis causes oedematous pale mucosa with abundant clear secretions from the lateral nasal wall where the narrow sinus outflow tracts of the OMC are found. This leads to decreased mucociliary clearance of the main sinus chambers and decreased sinus ventilation, predisposing to secondary bacterial sinusitis. On average, cilia do not recover normal function for 3 weeks.

Bacterial

Within the normal nasal and paranasal sinuses, bacterial flora include streptococci, staphylococci and corynebacteria. Bacterial rhinosinusitis is frequently secondary to an initiating viral infection. In acute bacterial rhinosinusitis, aerobic organisms are the main culprits, e.g. *Streptococcus pneumoniae*, *Haemophilus influenzae*, *Moraxella catarrhalis* and pneumococci.

In bacterial rhinosinusitis, the nasal mucosa is swollen, tender and coated with fibrin and mucopurulent secretions. Factors that may predispose to an infective rhinosinusitis include cigarette smoking and drugs that impede mucociliary transport.

Fungal sinusitis

There are four types. **Allergic fungal rhinosinusitis** (AFR) and the **saprophytic fungal ball** are non-invasive types with hyphae on the mucosa. Two **invasive** types with hyphae are found within the mucosa. **Chronic, indolent invasive disease** has a slow, erosive course. Patients may present with orbital proptosis following disease erosion into the orbital cavity. The **fulminant** type is angio-invasive with a rapid clinical course and occurs in the immunocompromised. AFR usually affects young adults and is invariably associated with nasal polyposis (NP). Between 5 and 10% of chronic rhinosinusitis (CRS) sufferers may really have AFR. Patients show elevated levels of IgE to one or more fungal antigens and a local eosinophilic host response to the presence of these fungi within the nose and paranasal sinuses.

Other factors (non-allergic, non-infective rhinosinusitis)

Non-allergic rhinitis with eosinophilia syndrome (NARES)

Eosinophilia is found in over 20% of patients with perennial nasal symptoms with no demonstrable allergy or cause for their disease. Eosinophils release proinflammatory mediators. Many patients are asthmatics.

Vasomotor rhinitis

This is often a diagnosis of exclusion, thought to be due to an imbalance of the autonomic nervous system, and so is better termed vasomotor instability. Parasympathetic action increases nasal gland secretion and congestion of nasal lining by altered vascular tone.

Hormonal rhinitis

Pregnancy, puberty, emotional changes and hypothyroidism are examples of causes of hormonal rhinitis.

Drug-induced rhinitis

Aspirin, oral contraceptives, high-dose oestrogen pills, beta blockers and angiotensin-converting enzyme (ACE) inhibitors are associated with nasal symptoms. Overuse of topical nasal decongestants may result in rebound congestion, nasal hyperreactivity, tolerance and histological changes – so-called rhinitis medicamentosa.

Rhinosinusitis with host defence deficiencies

Cystic fibrosis is an autosomal recessive disorder of exocrine glandular function, which manifests in the upper respiratory tract. There is thick mucus production that impairs mucociliary transport, so propagating infection.

A marked reduction in mucociliary beat frequency is known as primary ciliary dyskinesia. Conditions such as Kartagener's syndrome and Young's syndrome lead to poor mucociliary clearance and rhinosinusitis.

Granulomatous diseases such as sarcoidosis and Wegener's may present with lesions in the upper airways that cause crusting, obstruction and destruction of the nasal cavity.

Major immunoglobulin deficiency and IgG subclass deficiency also predispose to CRS.

Nasal polyposis

This is part of the spectrum of CRS. The prevalence of NP is 4% in the general population and is male predominated. It increases with age to a peak incidence in those aged 50 years or older. Up to 50% of NP patients have a family history.

No single predisposing disease is implicated in polyp formation, although NP is demonstrated in several diseases. The prevalence of NP increases to between 7 and 15% in patients with asthma.

Patients with nonsteroidal anti-inflammatory drug (NSAID) (salicylic acid) sensitivity are found to have between 36 and 60% prevalence of NP. Samter's triad describes a clinical syndrome of patients with asthma, aspirin/NSAID sensitivity and nasal polyps.

Nasal polyps are 'grape-like' bags of pale oedematous tissue, most commonly arising from the anterior ethmoid sinuses through the middle meatus into the nasal cavity (Fig. 9.4). Over time, squamous metaplasia occurs and they become fleshy and reddened. NPs are most commonly bilateral. There must be strong suspicion of neoplasia or fungal disease if unilateral polyps are found. Antrochoanal polyps are rare, and arise in the maxillary sinus with prolapse through the sinus ostium backwards into the nasopharynx. These are not thought to be inflammatory and do not respond to steroids.

There are links between systemic diseases and NP in cystic fibrosis and Kartagener's syndrome. Cystic fibrosis is the predominant cause of polyps in children and may be the first presenting problem.

Up to 80% of patients with NP demonstrate fungal growth on nasal swab culture, and approximately 30% of patients with NP have been found to have IgE antibodies to *Staphylococcus aureus* enterotoxins. These superantigens may be the stimulus for CRS and polyp formation.

Clinical presentation of paranasal sinus disease

Patients present with symptoms of:
- nasal blockage, congestion or stuffiness;
- nasal discharge or postnasal drip, which is often mucopurulent;
- facial pain and pressure with headache;
- reduction or loss of smell and taste.

They may also complain of associated symptoms such as a sore throat, dysphonia and cough with malaise and fever. Unilateral symptoms should always suggest neoplasm, particularly if accompanied by bloody discharge or facial pain.

A complete history should elicit details regarding the timescale of symptoms; seasonal or perennial cycles; trigger factors; family pets; effect on lifestyle; past medical history and drug history.

Examination

The nasal cavity is found to have a congested mucosal lining, which

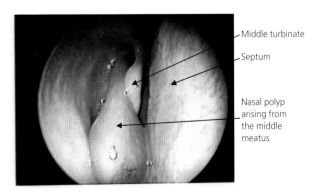

Figure 9.4 Nasal polyposis.

appears pink but, when grossly oedematous, will often be pale and boggy to palpate. Excessive mucus production with enlarged inferior turbinates and swollen anterior septal mucosa causes nasal airway congestion. Mucosal oedema in the lateral nasal wall and OMC may compromise sinus ventilation and drainage.

A large, swollen hypertrophied inferior turbinate is easily mistaken for a polyp. Polyps, though, are pale grey, translucent and lack any sensation to gentle palpation.

Sinonasal endoscopy enables an excellent view of the entire nasal cavity and lateral nasal wall, where early signs of polypoid or purulent sinusitis can be detected.

Differential diagnosis

Many patients suffer with midfacial pain incorrectly attributed to sinus disease; however, they may not have symptoms of nasal blockage, smell disturbance or nasal discharge.

Midfacial pain may be caused by migraine, tension headache or trigeminal neuralgia and hence the history is crucial to obtain a correct diagnosis.

Investigations

Allergy tests

Patients should be screened for airborne allergies to common pollens such as grass, trees and weeds, house dust mite and animal dander by skin prick testing (Fig. 9.5) when supported by the clinical history. Blood IgE levels may also contribute to an allergic diagnosis and are helpful in the presence of dermatographism.

Further blood tests

A full blood count will indicate levels of eosinophils. If concurrent systemic diseases are suspected, more complex tests for Wegener's granuloma and sarcoidosis should be performed. Immunoglobulin levels may also be measured.

Special tests

Nasal mucociliary clearance times may be measured using saccharine and, in specialist centres, nasal brushings for ciliary beat fre-

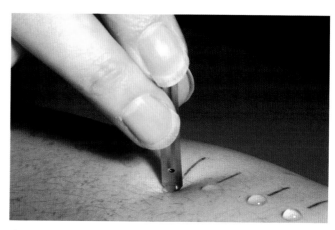

Figure 9.5 Skin prick allergy tests.

quency and cilia electron microscopy may be performed. Children with polyps should be tested for cystic fibrosis by sweat analysis and genotyping.

Imaging

Plain X-ray imaging is misleading, with poor sensitivity and specificity. It has no useful place in the diagnosis of chronic rhinosinusitis with or without polyposis.

Computed tomography (CT) of the sinuses in the coronal plane has become the international standard imaging method for staging disease (Fig. 9.6). Magnetic resonance imaging (MRI) is mainly used in the investigation of neoplasia or invasive fungal disease.

Complications of rhinosinusitis

Periorbital cellulitis may present with a unilateral orbital swelling with ophthalmoplegia and proptosis (Figs 9.7 and 9.8). An infective rhinosinusitis may breach the thin bone of the lamina papyracea and cause a subperiosteal abscess within the orbital cavity. If not treated urgently, this can spread further to penetrate the orbital cavity contents and cause an intraorbital abscess, thus endangering the optic nerve.

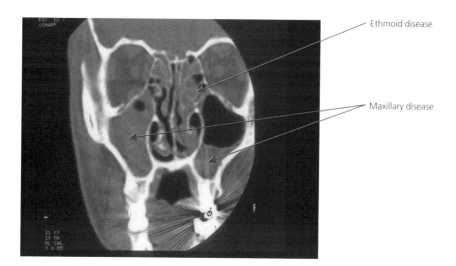

Ethmoid disease

Maxillary disease

Figure 9.6 Coronal CT image of rhinosinusitis.

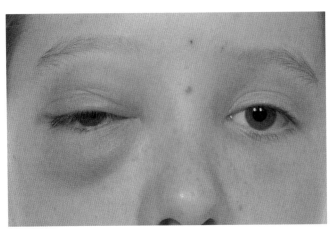

Figure 9.7 Right periorbital cellulitis secondary to infective rhinosinusitis.

Infective disease may also travel through the valveless venous plexus drainage passages of the paranasal sinuses to the cavernous sinus and cause a **cavernous sinus thrombosis**.

Frontal rhinosinusitis may rarely lead to osteomyelitis of the frontal bone that further disseminates to extradural, subdural and more rarely intradural abscess formation. Infection may also spread directly intracranially via thrombosed veins or through bony fissures. Metastatic intracerebral abscesses from sinusitis have been reported.

Treatment

See Figs 9.9–9.13 for algorithms and Boxes 9.1 and 9.2 for complications.

Surgery

Historically, nasal surgery was often performed under local anaesthetic, sparing general anaesthesia for more complex cases. Surgeons used snares and avulsing techniques to remove nasal polyps.

Maxillary sinuses were commonly washed out in the clinic, under local anaesthesia, for presumed infection by the passing of a tro-char under the inferior turbinate and through the thin medial wall of the maxillary sinus. Inferior meatal antrostomy might also be fashioned, creating a window into the antrum through the inferior meatus.

More extensive procedures using an external facial incision were employed to remove hyperplastic and polypoid sinus mucosa from frontal, maxillary and ethmoid sinuses and to create large, non-physiological drainage holes.

Current practice favours the use of functional endoscopic sinus surgery (FESS) tailored to the extent of disease demonstrated on the CT scan. The pre-chambers of the major sinuses in the OMC are cleared. This restores mucociliary clearance and ventilation through the natural ostia. Mucosa in the major sinuses may then return to normal precluding its exenteration. Polyps are removed to the extent of disease and normal mucosa is spared removal.

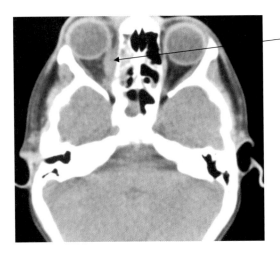

Subperiosteal abscess secondary to infective ethmoid rhinosinusitis

Figure 9.8 Axial CT scan.

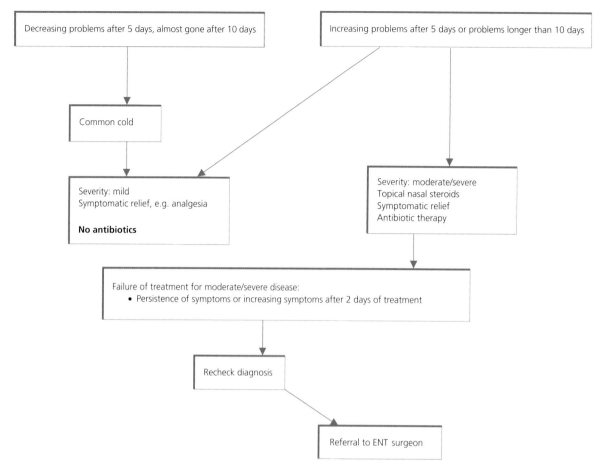

Figure 9.9 Algorithm 1 – acute rhinosinusitis.

Good illumination allows surgery to be performed through the nose avoiding facial incisions. Simple nasal polypectomy may be carried out to provide an airway. Even this conservative surgery benefits from better visualization.

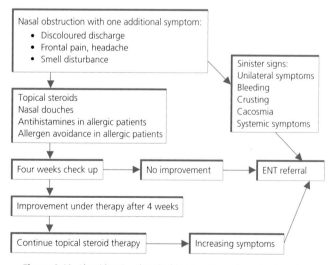

Figure 9.10 Algorithm 2 – chronic rhinosinusitis and nasal polyposis.

For severe disease, when landmarks may be distorted or absent, external approaches may still be employed but in combination with endoscopic intranasal approaches.

Complications of surgery

Minor complication rates are 1.44%, and major complication rates 0.44%.

Minor

- nasal adhesions
- epiphora
- black eye.

Major

- double vision
- partial or total loss of vision
- CSF leak
- meningitis
- cerebral injury
- intracranial bleed
- retrobulbar haemorrhage
- haemorrhage from internal carotid artery.

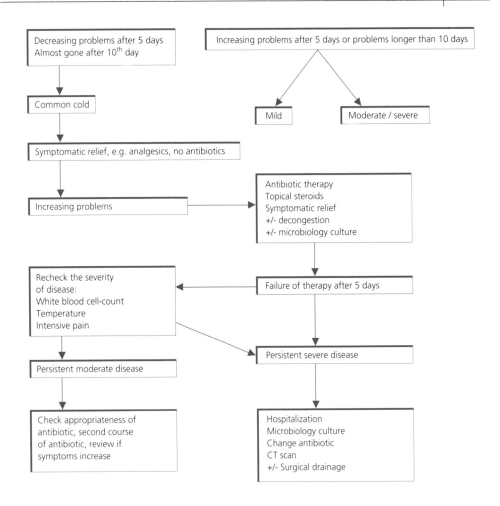

Figure 9.11 Algorithm 3 – ENT department treatment for acute rhinosinusitis.

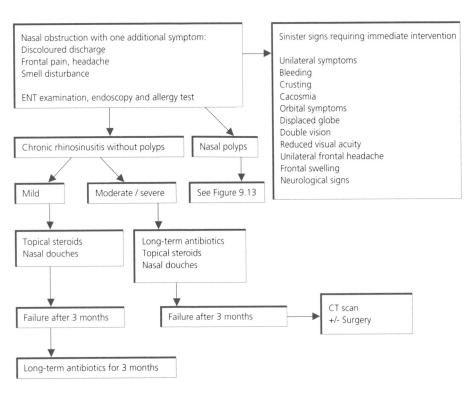

Figure 9.12 Algorithm 4 – ENT department treatment of chronic rhinosinusitis.

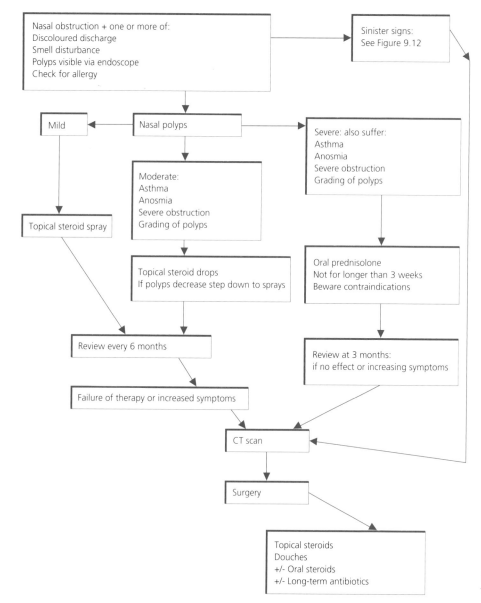

Figure 9.13 Algorithm 5 – ENT department treatment for nasal polyposis.

Further reading

Hadfield PJ, Rowe-Jones JM, Mackay IS. (2000) The prevalence of nasal polyps in adults with cystic fibrosis. *Clinical Otolaryngology*; 25(1): 19-22.

Hopkins C, Browne JP, Slack R *et al.* (2006) The national comparative audit of surgery for nasal polyposis and chronic rhinosinusitis. *Clinical Otolaryngology*; 31(5): 390–8.

Lund VJ, Hosemann W, Rowe-Jones J, Bitzer E, Jankowski R. (2004) Nasal surgery: evidence of efficacy. *Rhinology*; 42:246–54.

Rowe-Jones JM. (1998) Asthma, sinusitis and postnasal drip. *The Asthma Journal*; 63–7.

Rowe-Jones JM, Mackay IS. (1998) The management of nasal polyps. *Current Opinion in Otolaryngology & Head and Neck Surgery*; 6(1): 41-6.

Rowe-Jones J, Medcalf M, Durham S, Richards D, Mackay I. (2005) Functional Endoscopic Sinus Surgery: 5 year follow up and results of a prospective, randomised, stratified, double-blind, placebo controlled study of postoperative fluticasone propionate aqueous nasal spray. *Rhinology*; 43(1):2–10

Rowe-Jones JM, Wright D. (1994) Sinusitis: current treatment with functional endoscopic sinus surgery. *British Journal of Hospital Medicine*; 52(6): 269–74.

Further resources

www.aaaai.org
www.whiar.org
www.sinuseducation.org

CHAPTER 10

Facial Pain

Nick S Jones

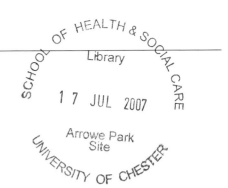
> **OVERVIEW**
>
> - If facial pain and pressure are the primary symptoms, the cause is unlikely to be sinus disease in the absence of any nasal symptoms or signs.
> - If a patient has facial pain as well as nasal obstruction and a loss of sense of smell, which is worse with the common cold or flying, then he or she is likely to be helped by nasal medical or, if that fails, surgical treatment.
> - Patients whose nasal endoscopy is normal are unlikely to have pain caused by rhinosinusitis.
> - Patients with a normal CT scan are unlikely to have pain due to rhinosinusitis (NB CT changes on their own are not indicative of symptomatic rhinosinusitis).
> - Patients with purulent secretions and facial pain are likely to benefit from treatment directed at resolving their rhinosinusitis.
> - If it is not possible to make a diagnosis at the first consultation, it is often helpful to ask the patient to keep a diary of his or her symptoms, carry out a trial of medical nasal treatment and review after this.

Most people are aware that the sinuses lie behind the facial bones; therefore, it is not surprising that many believe that the cause of their facial pain is their sinuses. However, rhinosinusitis is often not the cause of facial pain, even in an ENT clinic. It is important to get the diagnosis right in order to prevent the unnecessary prescription of antibiotics or sinus surgery.

A careful history is central for correct diagnosis. Examination is usually normal, but when there are neurological signs or evidence of purulent secretions this helps to make the diagnosis. Unrelated radiological findings are sufficiently common to limit the usefulness of computed tomography (CT) and magnetic resonance imaging (MRI) in the diagnosis of rhinosinusitis. If they are performed, any positive findings should be interpreted with caution in the light of the history and endoscopic findings.

Thirteen questions form the basis of a mental algorithm that will help you towards a diagnosis.

1 **Where is the pain?** Ask the patient to point to the site of the pain, not only because it locates it, but because the gesture often provides information about its nature and its emotional significance to the patient.

2 **How long is each episode?** A common misconception is that migraine only lasts a few hours, but it can last up to 48 hours.

3 **What treatment has been tried and with what effect?**

4 **How often does the pain occur?** The periodicity of symptoms may be a pointer to the diagnosis. For example, being woken in the morning by very severe facial pain suggests cluster headache.

5 **How did the pain begin?** Unilateral pain following a cold and associated with nasal obstruction and a persistent nasal discharge is indicative of infective rhinosinusitis.

6 **Is the pain continuous or intermittent?** Symmetrical pain persisting over weeks in the cheeks, behind the eyes, the bridge of the nose or affecting the forehead is more likely to be due to midfacial segment pain rather than rhinosinusitis.

7 **What is the pattern of the attacks and are they progressing?** A progressive headache associated with nausea or effortless vomiting means that an intracranial lesion should be excluded.

8 **What precipitates the pain?** Pain associated with clear exacerbating or relieving factors, whose onset is clear cut and whose site does not vary, usually has an organic cause.

9 **What relieves the pain?** Tension-type headache does not respond to analgesics, whereas patients with migraine often report that lying quietly in a dark room helps.

10 **Where is the pain and does it radiate anywhere?** Pain extending either across the midline or across neurological dermatomes is less likely to have a physical basis.

11 **Are there any associated symptoms?** Nausea accompanying the pain is characteristic, although not diagnostic, of migraine.

12 **What effect does it have on daily life and sleep?** Should the patient describe marked unrelenting pain, yet have a normal sleep pattern, atypical facial pain should be considered in the differential diagnosis.

13 **What type of pain is it?** A sensation of pressure is in keeping with tension-type headache or midfacial segment pain, whereas patients with migraine report a throbbing pain and a burning or gnawing pain is characteristic of neuropathic pain.

Facial pain often has some emotional significance. For some patients, facial pain may be greatly affected by emotional distress, anxiety or the psychological harm the patient associates with disease, trauma or surgery. It may sometimes be the means by which they obtain secondary gain. The presence of marked psychological overlay does not mean that there is no underlying organic problem, but it is a relative contraindication to surgical treatment. If there is a big discrepancy between the patient's affect and the description of the pain, the organic component of the illness may be of relatively minor importance. Should the diagnosis be elusive, re-taking the history at a further consultation may be helpful, as well as asking the patient to keep a symptom diary.

Tension-type headache

Tension-type headache has the qualities of tightness or pressure. It usually affects the forehead or temple, and often the suboccipital area as well (Fig. 10.1). It may be episodic or chronic (> 15 days per month, > 6 months), and is only occasionally helped by nonsteroidal anti-inflammatory drugs. Typically, patients take large quantities of analgesics yet say that they produce little benefit. Hyperaesthesia of the skin or muscles of the forehead often occurs, giving patients the impression they have rhinosinusitis, as they know their sinuses lie under the forehead. The majority of patients with this condition respond to low-dose amitriptyline, but they usually require up to 6 weeks of 10 mg and occasionally 20 mg at night before it works. Amitriptyline should then be continued for 6 months. Patients need to be warned of the sedative effects of even this low dose, but can be reassured that tolerance usually develops in the first few days. It is our practice to inform patients that amitriptyline is also used in higher doses for other conditions such as depression. If amitriptyline fails, then relief may be obtained from gabapentin.

Midfacial segment pain

This causes a symmetrical sensation of pressure or tightness across the middle third of the face, and it is not uncommon to have co-existing tension-type headache. The nature of midfacial segment pain is like tension-type headache, except that it affects the midface. Some patients, rather than describing symptoms of pressure, may say that the nose feels blocked, although they will have no nasal airway obstruction. These symptoms are often misinterpreted by the patient as sinusitis. The areas of pressure involve under the bridge of the nose, either side of the nose, the peri- or retro-orbital regions, or across the cheeks (Figs 10.2a–f). There may be hyperaesthesia of

the skin and soft tissues over the affected area on examination, and gently touching the affected area is enough to cause discomfort, whereas there is no evidence of underlying bony disease. Nasal endoscopy is normal. CT of the paranasal sinuses is normal.

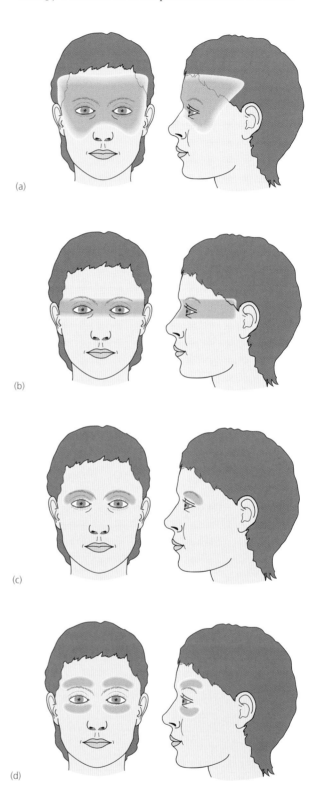

(a)

(b)

(c)

(d)

Figure 10.2 (a–f) Distribution of the symmetrical symptoms of pressure in midfacial segment pain. (*Continued*.)

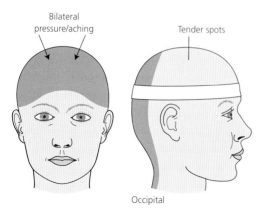

Figure 10.1 Diagrammatic representation of the features of tension-type headache.

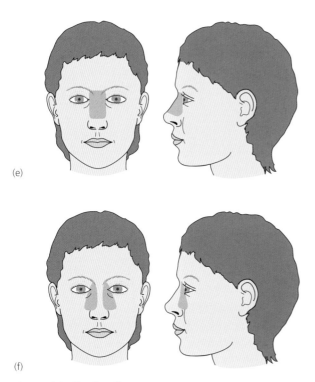

(e)

(f)

Figure 10.2 (Continued.)

Note that a third of asymptomatic patients have incidental mucosal changes on CT, and so radiographic changes are not diagnostic of rhinosinusitis (Marshall and Jones, 2003).

There is no consistent exacerbating or relieving factor. There are no real nasal symptoms (note that approximately 20% of most populations have intermittent or persistent allergic rhinitis, which may occur coincidentally in this condition).

Therefore, midfacial segment pain has all the characteristics of tension-type headache, with the exception that it affects the midface (West and Jones, 2001). Patients may have been treated over a long period with antibiotics and topical nasal steroids and some patients may have had some transient response on occasion, possibly related to the placebo effect or cognitive dissonance, but this is inconsistent.

The majority of patients with this condition respond to low-dose amitriptyline and are treated in the same way as patients with tension-type headache.

It seems likely that the underlying pathology in midfacial segment pain is similar to that in tension-type headache. The aetiology of this type of pain is uncertain, but Olesen's theory (Jensen and Olesen, 2000) that integrates the effects of myofascial afferents, the activation of peripheral nociceptors and their convergence on the caudal nucleus of the trigeminal nerve, along with qualitative changes in the central nervous system, provides one of the best models. There is also a suggestion that there is a downregulation of central inhibition from supraspinal impulses due to psychological stress and emotional disturbances. It is of interest that, if surgery is mistakenly performed as a treatment for midfacial segment pain, the pain may sometimes abate temporarily, only to return after several weeks to months.

Symmetrical facial pain involving the bridge of the nose, either side of the nose, behind the eyes, the supraorbital or infraorbital margins +/– the forehead is often due to midfacial segment pain.

Pain arising from the sinuses

Acute sinusitis usually follows an acute upper respiratory tract infection and pain is usually unilateral, intense, associated with fever and unilateral nasal obstruction, and there may be a purulent discharge. Chronic sinusitis is often painless, causing nasal obstruction due to mucosal hypertrophy, and with a purulent discharge that continues throughout the day (not just a collection in the morning that is usually due to postnasal mucus, stagnating in a mouth breather or snorer, that has become discoloured by local commensal organisms). An acute exacerbation can cause pain, but this rarely lasts for more than a few days. The pain is often a unilateral dull ache around the medial canthus of the eye, although more severe facial pain can occur, and in maxillary sinusitis toothache often occurs. An increase in the severity of pain on bending forward is traditionally thought to be diagnostic of sinusitis, but in fact many types of facial pain and headache are made worse by this action.

The key points in the history of sinogenic pain are an association with rhinological symptoms, and a response to medical treatment. Facial swelling is usually due to other pathology such as dental sepsis. If a diagnosis of sinusitis has been made and the patient has not responded to antibiotics, then nasendoscopy is very helpful, if not essential, in making or excluding the diagnosis of sinusitis. A normal nasal cavity, showing no evidence of middle meatal mucopus or inflammatory changes, makes a diagnosis of sinogenic pain most unlikely. Patients who report intermittent symptoms of facial pain can be asked to return for endoscopic examination when they are symptomatic (Hughes and Jones, 1998; Jones, 2004). In patients with genuine sinusitis, endoscopic sinus surgery has been shown to alleviate the facial pain in over 75% (Jones, 2004).

Facial pain without any nasal symptoms is unlikely to be due to sinusitis.

Proposed theories for the aetiology of rhinological pain

Some workers have put forward non-infective theories of facial pain, for example 'vacuum pain' and 'contact points'. Transient facial pain in patients with other symptoms and signs of rhinosinusitis can occur with pressure changes when flying, diving or skiing, but this resolves as the pressure within the sinuses equalizes through perfusion with the surrounding vasculature. The evidence that a vacuum within a blocked sinus can cause **protracted** pain is poor.

The theories that implicate contact points as a cause of facial pain have been questioned as the prevalence of contact points has been found to be the same in an asymptomatic population as in a symptomatic population, and when they were present in symptomatic patients with unilateral pain, they were present in the contralateral side to the pain in 50% of these patients (Abu-Bakra and Jones, 2001; Ahmed and Jones, 2003). Nowhere else in the body does mucosa–mucosa contact cause pain. Anatomical variations within the nose/sinuses have been said to be responsible for causing pain, but case-controlled studies have shown that these variations are as common in a symptomatic as an asymptomatic population (Marshall and Jones, 2003).

Pain following trauma or surgery

Occasionally following a nasal fracture, pain can persist over the nasal bridge. The cause of this is unclear and, whilst it is sometimes said to be due to a neuroma in the scar tissue, it appears to be influenced by the degree of distress the patient continues to feel about the insult he or she had received. It is possible that peripheral regenerative or deafferent changes may influence the trigeminal brain stem sensory nuclear complex, just as processes such as nerve compression, sympathetically mediated pain and neuroma formation can cause neuropathic pain (Sessle, 2000; Khan et al., 2002).

Migraine

Migraine causes severe headache, but in a small proportion of patients it can affect the cheek, orbit and forehead (Daudia and Jones, 2002). It is described as sharp, severe and throbbing and is invariably accompanied by nausea. Premenstruation, diet, stress or stress withdrawal can induce an attack, as with classical migraine. There is often a family history of migraine.

Cluster headache

Cluster headache typically presents with a very severe unilateral stabbing or burning pain, which may be frontal, temporal, ocular, over the cheek, or even in the maxillary teeth (Fig. 10.3). There is often rhinorrhoea, unilateral nasal obstruction, lacrimation and sometimes conjunctival infection. It is most common in men between the ages of 30 and 50 years. The patient is awakened in the early hours, often walking around the bedroom in distress, with the pain lasting between 30 minutes and 2 hours, and myosis or facial flushing may be seen. It may be precipitated by alcohol intake.

Chronic paroxysmal hemicrania

Chronic paroxysmal hemicrania is an excruciating pain occurring in women at any time of the night or day. It can affect the frontal, ocular, cheek or temporal regions and lasts from 30 minutes to 3 hours. The patient can experience several episodes in 24 hours and nasal congestion, lacrimation and facial flushing can all be a feature.

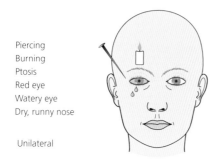

Piercing
Burning
Ptosis
Red eye
Watery eye
Dry, runny nose

Unilateral

Figure 10.3 The features of cluster headache.

Eye-related pain

Uncorrected optical refractive errors can cause headaches, but their importance is exaggerated. Pain on ocular movement is suggestive of optic neuritis or scleritis. It is vital to recognize acute glaucoma that may cause severe orbital pain and headache. The patient may see haloes around lights, and may feel very unwell with vomiting. The eye may show signs of circumcorneal infection. Orbital pain can also be caused by uveitis, keratitis and dry eye syndrome. Disease involving the optic nerve results in reduced acuity and colour vision. Testing visual acuity is important in assessing intraocular disease and, if it is abnormal with the patient's glasses (if they are used), an ophthalmological opinion is needed.

Teeth, jaws and related structures

All too often pain in the upper jaw is thought to be of dental or sinus origin, and it may not be until several extractions or sinus surgical procedures have been performed without benefit that it becomes apparent that the pain was and is neurological and is often due to 'phantom tooth pain'. It is important not to perform surgery or extract teeth without good objective evidence that they are the cause.

Temporomandibular joint dysfunction is most commonly unilateral (90%) and usually occurs in young adults with a history of bruxism, clenching, trauma, recent dental work, anxiety, enthusiastic kissing, or cradling the telephone between the jaw and the shoulder. Pain is caused by pterygoid spasm and is described as a deep, dull ache that may masquerade as toothache or earache. There is often a superimposed sharper component that may radiate down the jaw, or over the side of the face or temple. Clicking of the temporomandibular joint is an unreliable sign, whereas trismus and deviation of the jaw from the midline on opening help confirm the diagnosis; there may be tenderness of the joint on palpation.

Trigeminal neuralgia

Trigeminal neuralgia is more common in women over 40 years of age, with a peak incidence between 50 and 60 years. Patients complain of paroxysms of agonizing, lancinating pain induced by a specific trigger point, although there is a refractory period of more than 30 seconds. In more than a third of sufferers, the pain occurs in both the maxillary and mandibular divisions, whilst in a fifth it is confined to the mandibular region and in 3% to the ophthalmic division. Typical trigger sites are the lips and the nasolabial folds, but pain may also be triggered by touching the gingivae. Remissions are common but it is not unusual for the attacks to increase in frequency and severity. Beware the dental pain that can mimic trigeminal neuralgia, particularly a fractured tooth, or exposed cervical dentine. In patients under 40 years old, it is most commonly due to multiple sclerosis.

Atypical facial pain

This is a diagnosis of exclusion and it is important to exclude organic disease. The history is often vague or inconsistent with widespread pain extending from the face to other areas of the head and neck. Pain is typically deep and ill defined, changes location, is unexplainable on an anatomical basis, occurs almost daily and is sometimes fluctuating, sometimes continuous, has no precipitating factors and is not relieved by analgesics. Specific questioning about the symptoms often results in vague answers. The pain does not wake the patient up, and although the patient reports that her or she cannot sleep, he or she will often look well rested. It is more common in women over the age of 40. There may be a history of other pain syndromes and the patient's extensive records show minimal progress despite various medications. Many patients with atypical facial pain exhibit evidence of psychological disturbance or a history of depression and are unable to function normally as a result of their pain. The management of such patients is challenging and confrontation is nearly always counterproductive. A good starting point is to reassure the patients that you recognize that they have genuine pain, and an empathetic consultation with an explanation should be conducted. Drug treatment revolves around a gradual build-up to the higher analgesic and antidepressant levels of amitriptyline (75–100 mg) at night.

Headache and sinusitis

Patients with facial pain or headache without nasal symptoms are very unlikely to be helped by nasal medical or surgical treatment.

Conclusions

The majority of patients who present with facial pain and headaches believe they have 'sinus trouble'. There is an increasing awareness amongst otorhinolaryngologists that neurological causes are responsible for a large proportion of headache and facial pain (West and Jones, 2001). We believe that patients with facial pain who have no objective evidence of sinus disease (endoscopy negative) are unlikely to be helped by nasal medical or surgical treatment. In these patients, other diagnoses should be considered and appropriate medical treatment tried.

A comprehensive examination including nasendoscopy is highly desirable if medical nasal treatment directed at sinusitis has failed, in order to confirm or refute the diagnosis of sinusitis.

Further reading

Abu-Bakra M, Jones NS. (2001) The prevalence of nasal contact points in a population with facial pain and a control population. *Journal of Laryngology and Otology*; **115**: 629–32.

Ahmed S, Jones NS. (2003) What is Sluder's neuralgia? *Journal of Laryngology and Otology*; **117**: 437-43.

Daudia A, Jones NS. (2002) Facial migraine in a rhinological setting. *Clinical Otolaryngology*; **27**: 521–5.

Hughes R, Jones NS. (1998) The role of endoscopy in outpatient management. *Clinical Otolaryngology*; **23**: 224–6.

Jensen R, Olesen J. (2000) Tension-type headache: an update on mechanisms and treatment. *Current Opinion in Neurology*; **13**: 285–9.

Jones NS. (2004) Midfacial segment pain: implications for rhinitis and sinusitis. *Current Allergy and Asthma Reports*; **4**: 187–92.

Khan O, Majumdar S, Jones NS. (2002) Facial pain after sinus surgery and trauma. *Clinical Otolaryngology*; **27**: 171–4.

Marshall A, Jones NS. (2003) The utility of radiological studies in the diagnosis and management of rhinosinusitis. *Current Infectious Diseases Reports*; **5**: 199–204.

Scully C, Felix DH. (2006). Oral Medicine: Orofacial pain. *British Dental Journal*; **200**: 75–80.

Sessle BJ. (2000) Acute and chronic craniofacial pain: brainstem mechanisms of nociceptive transmission and neuroplasticity, and other clinical correlates. *Critical Reviews in Oral Biology & Medicine*; **11**(1): 57–91.

West B, Jones NS. (2001) Endoscopy-negative, computed tomography-negative facial pain in a nasal clinic. *Laryngoscope*; **111**: 581–6.

CHAPTER 11

Sore Throats

William McKerrow, Patrick J Bradley

OVERVIEW

- A sore throat as a presenting symptom to a general practitioner is very common. The majority of such symptoms are due to viral infections with symptoms that last for a few days, and most will respond to simple analgesics.

- A bacterial infection generally presents with soreness, otalgia and dysphagia with systemic upset and pyrexia, and requires analgesia as well as antibiotics for 7+ days.

- Indication for tonsillectomy currently remains controversial, but, when performed, great symptomatic relief is reported by the majority of patients.

- Complications, such as peritonsillar and parapharyngeal abscess, must be considered when symptoms are not resolving quickly, and specialist referral is to be encouraged.

- Sore throat with airway distress must be considered very serious and, when encountered, patients of whatever age should be referred to hospital, to ensure that an airway is maintained, and appropriate treatment with fluid replacement, antibiotics and possibly surgery is available with urgency should the scenario deteriorate suddenly.

- Chronic sore throat is seldom due to bacteria, and rarely if ever responds to courses of antibiotics. Other causes need to be excluded, such as cancers and specific infections which may require examination under anaesthetic. Referral should be considered if such symptoms persist for several weeks without a specific diagnosis.

Throat symptoms

Symptoms affecting the throat are very common, especially in children. The most common symptom is one of soreness or pain, which can vary in severity and periodicity. Pain is usually related to activity of and/or infections in the lymphoid tissue surrounding the upper airway (Waldeyer's ring), consisting of paired lingual and pharyngeal tonsils, as well as the adenoids that are placed behind the soft palate. There is overlap between pharyngitis and tonsillitis and between bacterial and viral infections, which cannot be reliably differentiated clinically. Bacteria are the primary pathogens identified in less than a third of cases.

Presentation

Relevant factors in the history include duration, severity (including

presence of systemic upset and neck lymphadenopathy), history of previous episodes and response to antibiotics. Symptoms localized to one side may indicate peritonsillar abscess (quinsy; see below). Referred pain to the ear is common, and sore throat radiating to the ear raises a possibility of neoplasm, particularly in older patients. Other causes of sore throat include infectious mononucleosis and rare conditions such as vasculitis, agranulocytosis and neoplasms, as well as complications of tonsillitis including deep neck space abscess. Sore throat, which may be associated with a potential airway obstruction, can present and affect all patient age groups, as the cause and source of the obstruction may be located at the epiglottis and the supraglottis.

Patients presenting with difficulty breathing, with severe systemic symptoms or with external swelling in the neck should be referred urgently.

Diagnosis and treatment

In most cases, the diagnosis of acute sore throat is straightforward, and symptomatic management with analgesia and gargles is all that is required. Antibiotic use in sore throat is controversial, as is the place for tonsillectomy.

There are no clinical or laboratory tests that reliably differentiate bacterial from viral sore throat quickly enough to help the general practitioner. Throat swabs may grow pathogenic bacteria, including beta haemolytic streptococci, even if the infection is primarily viral, and rapid antigen testing has variable specificity and sensitivity. The more reliable anti-streptolysin O titre is not usually available in time to inform treatment.

Antibiotics may reduce the incidence of the septic complications of tonsillitis, such as otitis media, sinusitis and peritonsillar abscess, and shorten the duration of the illness somewhat. This modest benefit needs to be balanced against the adverse effects of diarrhoea, skin rashes and (rarely) severe allergic reaction. There is also the danger of encouraging antibiotic-resistant organisms.

It is wise to manage most sore throats without antibiotics, apart from those with severe systemic upset or worsening symptoms. Penicillin V remains the drug of choice with erythromycin for those who are penicillin allergic and cephalosporins as an alternative. Amoxycillin and its derivatives should be avoided because of the risk of severe skin rashes in unsuspected infectious mononucleosis.

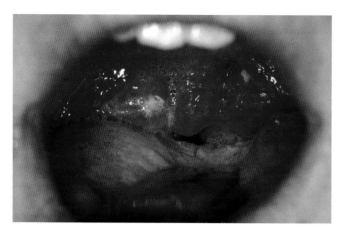

Figure 11.1 Acute tonsillitis.

Indications for tonsillectomy

Indications for tonsillectomy have become more stringent recently, with a reduction in numbers as risk/benefit analysis has developed (Fig. 11.1). There is also a better understanding of the natural history, at least in children with relatively mild symptoms who are likely to improve over 3 years. Tonsillectomy is reasonable if the infection is due to true tonsillitis, is severe enough to preclude normal activity and has been recurring on and off for at least a year, with at least five episodes. The benefits must be balanced against a small but significant risk of complications, particularly haemorrhage, which had an incidence of 2–8% in one national audit.

The incidence of surgery diminishes with age, particularly over 30. There is a distinct group of adults with low-grade continuing sore throat symptoms, punctuated by occasional acute episodes due to chronic tonsil sepsis, who may be helped by tonsillectomy.

Sore throats with cervical adenopathy

Severe sore throat with marked neck lymphadenopathy in young people, particularly with no history of recurrent sore throat, may be due to infectious mononucleosis, and the monospot test should be checked in these cases. Management is supportive, but severe cases may need admission for intravenous rehydration. Antibiotics, and sometimes steroids, are usually given in hospital despite the viral cause, as secondary bacterial infection, sometimes with anaerobes, is common. Epstein–Barr virus is the most common cause, although cytomegalovirus, toxoplasmosis, rubella and human immunodeficiency virus (HIV) are also implicated. During recovery, patients should be warned to avoid contact sports for at least 6 weeks because of a risk of damage to an enlarged liver and spleen, and abnormal liver function should be monitored until recovery is complete.

Complications of throat sepsis

Quinsy

Peritonsillar abscess (quinsy) presents as a unilateral erythematous swelling lateral to the tonsil, and in a patient with systemic upset is the commonest septic complication. Restricted mouth opening is usual. Traditional management by incision in the unanaesthetized patient (topical anaesthesia being potentially dangerous because of the risk of aspiration of pus) has been replaced by aspiration with a large-bore hypodermic needle. Antibiotics, usually penicillin V, with or without metronidazole are administered.

Parapharyngeal abscess

Deep neck space infection secondary to tonsil, or sometimes dental, sepsis is less common, but needs management in hospital, sometimes with airway protection by intubation or tracheostomy before surgical incision and drainage and infusion of intravenous antibiotics (see Fig. 11.2). The commonest variety is parapharyngeal abscess presenting in a severely ill patient with marked unilateral, tender, often red, neck swelling.

Acute retropharyngeal abscess

This is uncommon and usually secondary to tonsil or adenoid sepsis, sometimes in the immune compromised (Fig. 11.3). Airway protection before incision and drainage, which may be peroral, is essential. Tuberculosis is a rare cause for chronic retropharyngeal abscess nowadays in Western countries, but needs to be excluded.

Sore throat with acute airway distress

Acute upper airway distress or obstruction is most commonly inflammatory (Fig. 11.4), usually due to bacterial infection with *Haemophilus influenzae*. Vaccination programmes have reduced the incidence of this once common paediatric illness, usually manifesting as acute epiglottitis, but it is still seen quite commonly in adults where the infection tends to affect the whole supraglottic region. Mild cases in cooperative adults may be investigated by nasopharyngeal endoscopy, but there is a risk, particularly in children, of precipitating complete airway obstruction, and interference of any kind should be avoided – even the use of a tongue depressor or attempts at imaging. Large doses of intravenous broad-spectrum antibiotics, usually a third generation cephalosporin, with intravenous steroids are the management of choice and will usually result in improvement if not complete resolution within 48–72 hours.

The life-threatening nature of this disease cannot be over-emphasized. Rapid deterioration, even in apparently stable patients, may occur to precipitate critical airway obstruction.

Sore throat with subacute airway obstruction

In adults, subacute stridor may be caused by neoplasia, most commonly in the subglottic region (see Chapter 19), or rarely due to bilateral vocal cord palsy from neurological disease, or may be a complication of thyroid neoplasia or surgery.

Sore throat with a chronic upper airway obstruction

Low-grade upper airway obstruction in adults may be due to neoplasms or rarer conditions such as amyloidosis, sarcoid or vascu-

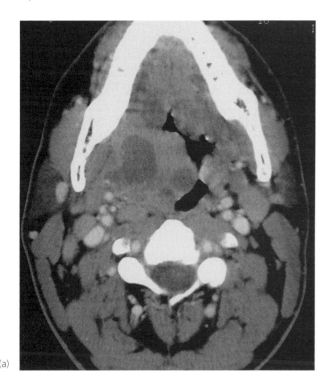

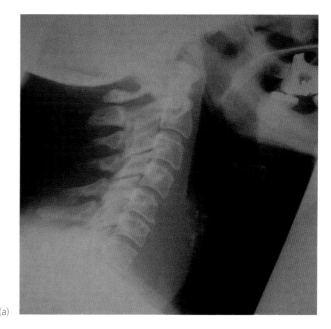

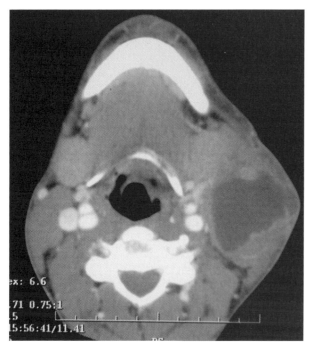

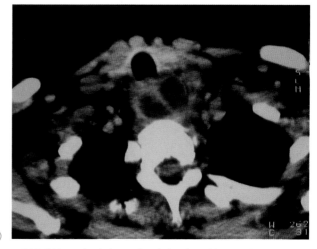

Figure 11.3 (a) Lateral soft tissue of neck showing widening of retropharyngeal space and (b) CT scan of the same patient showing abscess cavity in retropharyngeal space.

Figure 11.2 (a) Tonsillar and parapharyngeal abscess and (b) large neck abscess secondary to tonsillitis.

Pharyngitis

Pharyngitis may be acute and is most often caused by viruses, rhinoviruses, influenza A and B, herpes simplex and zoster and other infections involving pharyngeal lymphoid tissue. The symptoms of pharyngitis may not correlate with the clinical picture on inspection.

Chronic pharyngitis may be specific or non-specific. Non-specific pharyngitis is more difficult to define and diagnose. Patients usually complain of long-standing discomfort in the throat, pain or catching on swallowing, and sometimes earache. The observation of red patches on the posterior pharyngeal wall is not a reliable indication for a firm diagnosis, nor are there any helpful laboratory tests. There are a number of sources of infection of the lymphoid tissue of

litis, notably Wegener's granuloma. Patients present with noisy breathing or hoarseness and may be distressed or cyanosed. They should be referred early for specialist care. Examination with the flexible nasolaryngoscope is the first step, followed up by endoscopy and biopsy under general anaesthesia when appropriate (Fig. 11.5).

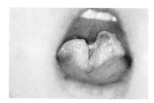

Figure 11.4 Rare case of diphtheria oropharyngitis.

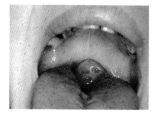

Figure 11.5 Lingual tonsillar tissue which may present with chronic upper airway obstruction.

the posterior pharyngeal wall – chronic sinusitis with postnasal pus irritation from above, chronic bronchitis and bronchiectasis from the respiratory tract below, as well as laryngo-pharyngeal reflux from the upper gastrointestinal system. Local irritants from tobacco, alcohol or industrial fumes are possible causes. Referral is indicated to exclude patients with primary pharyngeal carcinoma. Chronic pharyngitis is expressed by the patient as 'soreness in the throat', sometimes associated with catarrh. It is rarely associated with pyrexia or systemic upset. Rarely, if ever, will this symptom respond to antibiotics, and they should **not** be given as they are ineffective and may result in the development of resistance or side effects. Chronic specific pharyngitis may be associated with specific bacterial organisms: syphilis, tuberculosis, toxoplasmosis, leprosy, and scleroma. These are recognized by a localized physical abnormality, followed by biopsy and culture of the tissue. Specific treatment usually resolves the infection, but patients may remain symptomatic from scarring of local tissues.

Oral mucosal lesions

Mucosal abnormalities generally take the form of altered colour – generalized redness, or white or red patches. Ulcerative defects, swellings and occasionally papillomatous lesions also occur. Some common lesions may be identified from appearance alone, but many require biopsy for diagnosis, which may usually be achieved under local anaesthesia.

Inflammation

Acute inflammation of the oral cavity mucosa may arise from contact with irritants, or allergic responses to foodstuffs. Peanut allergy in children and young adults is increasingly common and manifests as irritation and swelling of the lips and oral mucosa. Progression to airway obstruction can develop. Prompt hospital treatment with antihistamine and intravenous steroids is essential to abort this potential danger.

Chronic inflammation of the oral mucosa follows ingestion of irritants (spices, spirits or heavy tobacco use), and may eventually progress to neoplasia. Inflammation also arises from irritation by rough, irregular teeth or ill-fitting dentures.

Candidal or fungal infection is commonly seen in the oral cavity of the elderly, and may manifest as redness and soreness of the mouth, sometimes with angular chelitis. Frequent recurrent fungal infections can occur, and are most commonly seen in denture wearers as prosthetic teeth can harbour the candidal organisms. Other patients who may present with fungal infections are those on steroid inhalers for chronic respiratory airway diseases, and also patients who are immunocompromised. Severe cases exhibit white plaques on the oral mucosa, commonly on the soft palate, but frequently generalized redness is the only evidence. Culture is diagnostic but the swab must be taken by vigorous rubbing of the tongue if it is to yield a positive result. Prolonged treatment with nystatin or clotrimazole, and occasionally with a systemic antifungal agent, is required for eradication. Dentures should be sterilized daily to prevent reinfection.

Ulceration

Ulceration commonly occurs in the form of **aphthous ulcers** (Fig. 11.6), which are painful and self-limiting in the course of about 10 days. They have a well-demarcated edge with a white sloughy base and are usually a few millimetres in diameter. Management is with topical pain-relieving medication such as 'Bonjela' (cetalkonium & choline salicylate) or 'Difflam' (benzydamine hydrochloride). Referral is advisable for further patient management. Topical steroid preparations are available and may help to provide symptomatic relief. Occasionally, ulcers are larger and more painful and persistent, in the condition known as **major aphthi**. The cause is unknown.

Oral ulceration is occasionally seen in serious systemic disease such as agranulocytosis and vasculitic disorders, and oral mucosal changes may occur as the manifestation of HIV in the form of 'hairy leucoplakia'. The typical 'punched out' ulcer of primary syphilis of the oral cavity is now relatively rare in the developed world, but

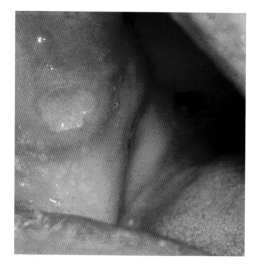

Figure 11.6 Aphthous ulcer.

should be considered as part of the differential diagnosis. The benign incidental finding of 'geographical tongue' is often mistaken for oral ulceration, but is in fact a normal variant. Many of these conditions and lesions may affect the posterior tongue and, unless diagnosed early, patients may try all remedies that are available 'over the counter' (and ultimately may become a clinical nuisance).

Neoplasia

Field change of the oral mucosa ranging from chronic inflammation through mild to severe dysplasia is common in association with heavy tobacco and alcohol usage, particularly in combination, and may progress via carcinoma *in situ* to frank squamous carcinoma. Any persistent white or red patches in the oral cavity, particularly in areas directly exposed to high concentrations of smoke and particularly dark spirits, should be regarded as suspicious and submitted to biopsy. Leucoplakia is easily confused with lichen planus, which is typified by a lacy white pattern on the mucosa, particularly in the buccal region.

Carcinomatous change is discussed in Chapter 19.

Further reading

Del Mar CB, Glasziou PP, Spinks AB. (2004) Antibiotics for sore throat. *The Cochrane Database of Systematic Reviews*, **2**, CD000023; DOI: 10.1002/14651858.CD000023.pub2

Katori H, Tsukuda M. (2005) Acute epiglottis: Analysis of factors associated with Airway Intervention. *Journal of Laryngology and Otology*; **119**: 967–72.

Mckerrow WS. Tonsillitis. *BMJ Clinical Evidence*, www.clinicalevidence.com

van Staaij BK, van den Akker EH, Rovers MM *et al.* (2004) Effectiveness of adenotonsillectomy in children with mild symptoms of throat infections or adenotonsillar hypertrophy: open, randomised controlled trial. *British Medical Journal*; **329**: 651–4.

Ridder GJ, Technau-Ihling K, Sander A, Boedeker CC. (2005) Spectrum and Management of Deep Neck Space Infections: An 8 year Experience of 234 cases. *Otolaryngol Head Neck Surg*; **133**: 709–14.

Scully C, Felix DH. (2005) Oral Medicine: Aphthous and other common ulcers. *British Dental Journal*; **199**: 259 –64.

Scully C, Felix DH. (2005) Oral Medicine: Mouth Ulcers of more serious connotation. *British Dental Journal*; **199**: 339 – 343.

CHAPTER 12

Breathing Disorders

Vinidh Paleri, Patrick J Bradley

> **OVERVIEW**
>
> - Stridor is a symptom NOT a diagnosis, and always requires examination and investigation. It denotes a harsh, vibratory noise from turbulent flow through a partially obstructed segment of respiratory tract.
> - All patients presenting with stridor, acute or chronic, must be investigated urgently.
> - The prime aim of managing a patient with stridor is to establish a secure and stable airway by intubation or tracheostomy.

Pathophysiology

Breathing is involuntarily controlled by the respiratory centre in the brain stem. The vocal cords abduct during inspiration and, with the negative pressure caused by diaphragmatic contraction and expansion of the chest, air is drawn into the lungs. The recurrent laryngeal branches of the vagus nerves control vocal cord movement, with intrinsic laryngeal muscles providing fine control. The cricoid cartilage is the only complete ring in the respiratory tract, surrounding the subglottic region. Any airway oedema there reduces its lumen. One millimetre of mucosal oedema reduces the cross-sectional area by more than 40%.

Stridor is a harsh, vibratory noise from turbulent flow through a partially obstructed segment of the respiratory tract. This is differentiated from **stertor**, where noise is caused by vibration of pharyngeal structures, leading to a lower pitched sound. Stridor can be present during the inspiratory or the expiratory phase or be biphasic (Box 12.1).

Stridor in children

Evaluation

History provides pointers to the diagnosis (Box 12.2). A previously

---

> Box 12.1 **Types of stridor**
>
> - Inspiratory: supraglottic and glottic obstruction.
> - Expiratory: low tracheal obstruction.
> - Biphasic: glottic and subglottic obstruction.

> Box 12.2 **Historical information**
>
> - Age of onset
> - Duration/phase of stridor
> - Worsening/improvement of stridor since onset
> - Precipitating causes
> - Failure to gain weight
> - Breath-holding spells
> - Fever
> - Feeding/swallowing problems
> - Hoarse/muffled voice
> - Intubation in the past
> - Cough/chest infections

---

well child presenting with acute onset stridor arouses suspicion of **foreign body aspiration**. Preceding upper respiratory tract infection (URTI) indicates **croup** or **bacterial tracheitis**. **Epiglottitis (supraglottitis)** typically presents as rapid onset fever, dysphagia and drooling in children from 2 to 7 years old.

A child with acute stridor must be assessed where instrumentation and experienced personnel are available for emergency intervention to protect the airway. Clinical assessment is shown in Box 12.3. Respiratory rate and level of consciousness are the most important indicators of severity of obstruction. Intensity of the sound does not indicate severity, as severe obstruction so reduces airflow that stridor is inaudible. **The child must not be upset in case of precipitating acute obstruction**.

> Box 12.3 **Clinical evaluation**
>
> - Respiratory rate
> - Cyanosis
> - Apnoeic spells
> - Use of accessory muscles
> - Intercostal/sternal retraction
> - Nasal flaring
> - Timing/severity of stridor
> - Hoarseness
> - Temperature/toxicity
> - Level of consciousness
> - ENT examination in controlled setting

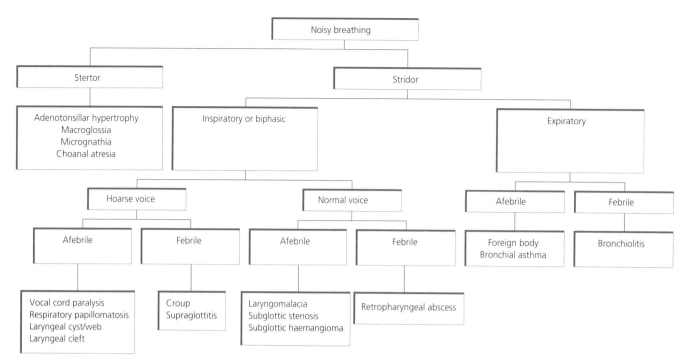

Figure 12.1 Differential diagnosis of stridor in children.

The probable cause is usually surmised before direct examination (Fig. 12.1). Most conditions are evolving when first seen, and observation needs intensive care or a high dependency setting.

Congenital structural lesions rarely present acutely. Chronic stridor usually needs diagnostic laryngotracheoscopy unless mild and easily diagnosed on clinical examination alone. In a cooperative child with no evidence of hypoxia, flexible laryngoscopy in the clinic can be very informative.

Acute stridor
Epiglottitis (supraglottitis)
Haemophilus influenzae **type B** is the usual infective agent. Incidence has decreased with HiB vaccination. Children between 2 and 7 years are affected, with peak incidence at 3. The disease presents with rapid onset of high fever, toxicity, agitation, stridor, dyspnoea, muffled voice and painful swallowing. The child sits leaning forward with mouth open and drooling. If epiglottitis is suspected, no further examination should be performed outside a controlled setting. The risk of complete obstruction is high. Endotracheal intubation is preferred as the supraglottic swelling usually subsides in a few days. A swollen, cherry red epiglottis is seen on direct laryngoscopy. Intravenous antibiotics are essential.

Laryngotracheobronchitis
The most common cause of acute stridor in childhood is laryngotracheobronchitis or 'croup'. **Parainfluenza virus** is the commonest cause, with influenza virus types A or B, respiratory syncytial virus and rhinoviruses sometimes being implicated. Children between 6 months and 3 years are affected, with peak incidence at 2. Symptoms include low-grade fever, barking cough, inspiratory

stridor and hoarseness, worse at night and aggravated by crying. No endoscopy is needed. Nebulized epinephrine with intravenous steroids is recommended. Rarely, intubation and ventilation are necessary.

Acute retropharyngeal and peritonsillar abscesses
Drooling, painful swallowing and systemic upset are usually seen at presentation, usually with a preceding URTI. Retropharyngeal abscesses in the lower pharynx may cause stridor, neck stiffness and torticollis. A soft tissue lateral X-ray of the neck shows diagnostic widening of the space between the vertebral column and the airway. Peritonsillar abscesses cause trismus and stertor. Urgent drainage is required.

Chronic stridor
Gastro-oesophageal reflux is a problem in children with chronic stridor – in up to 80% of cases. This is caused by the strong thoraco-abdominal pressure gradient of airway obstruction.

Laryngomalacia
This accounts for 75% of all causes of stridor in infants. **Weakness** of the supraglottic structures leads to prolapse of the supraglottis during inspiration (Figs 12.2 and 12.3). It presents as inspiratory or variable stridor between the fourth and sixth weeks of life. Stridor is worsened by crying and feeding and is relieved in the prone position. It is a self-limiting condition.

Subglottic stenosis
This may be **congenital** or **iatrogenic** (secondary to prolonged intubation and ventilation) (Fig. 12.4). Symptoms include inspiratory or biphasic stridor, usually in the first year of life. Iatrogenic stenosis

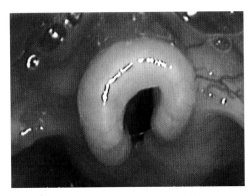

Figure 12.2 Laryngomalacia showing open airway during expiration (Courtesy Dr H. Kubba).

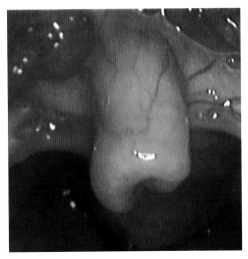

Figure 12.3 Laryngomalacia showing epiglottic collapse during inspiration (Courtesy Dr H. Kubba).

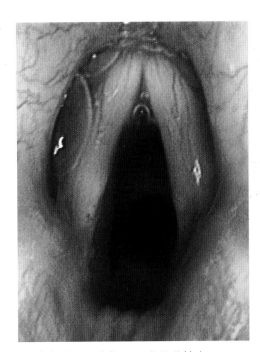

Figure 12.4 Subglottic stenosis (Courtesy Dr H. Kubba).

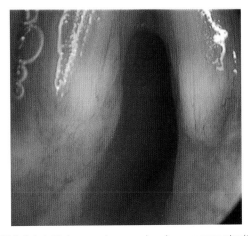

Figure 12.5 Subglottic haemangioma causing airway compromise (Courtesy Dr H. Kubba).

is suspected if stridor presents after extubation. Mild stenoses can be observed during laryngeal growth. Surgical reconstruction may be needed.

Vocal cord paralysis

This is usually met within the first month of life with stridor, cyanosis, apnoea and feeding problems. Concomitant **neurological disease**, such as hydrocephalus and Arnold-Chiari malformation, is present in most patients. Diagnosis is established by rigid endoscopy and assessment of vocal cord mobility. Management depends upon severity and progression. Spontaneous recovery may take up to 3 years. Tracheostomy may be needed.

Subglottic haemangioma

A **capillary haemangioma** in the subglottis presents between 6 weeks and 6 months of life (Fig. 12.5). Cutaneous haemangiomas offer a hint to the diagnosis. Intermittent stridor and a tendency to recurrent episodes of 'croup' are typical. Haemangiomas may grow for a year, followed by spontaneous regression, so they can be observed. A tracheostomy may be needed until regression. Other

treatment options include laser vaporization, excision and systemic steroids.

Respiratory papillomatosis

This is caused by the **human papilloma virus**. Transmission can occur from the mother to the child during labour. Hoarse voice is the usual presenting symptom, and the airway may be compromised. Stridor may need urgent debulking of the papillomatous lesions (Fig. 12.6). Tracheostomy should be avoided as this may provoke spread of papillomas into the lower airways. Resolution usually occurs during adolescence. Regular surveillance is needed with debulking or vaporization by a laser as necessary. Addition of topical cidofovir (an antiviral agent) reduces recurrences.

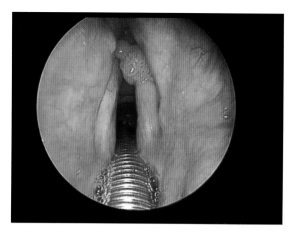

Figure 12.6 Papilloma on the right true vocal cord.

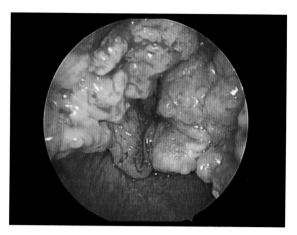

Figure 12.7 Laryngeal cancer causing complete obstruction of the glottis with superficial bleeding caused by intubation.

Evaluation of stridor in adults

Without definite precipitating cause or relevant history, acute and chronic stridor in adults should be considered neoplastic unless proven otherwise. A careful history may indicate causes such as previous thyroid surgery (bilateral recurrent laryngeal nerve injury) and intubation trauma. Assessment of the extent of hypoxia and the work of breathing is described in Boxes 12.2 and 12.3. It is possible to assess the larynx with a flexible nasolaryngoscope and to achieve a diagnosis in the outpatient setting in most adults.

Bilateral vocal cord palsy

The commonest cause of this condition used to be thyroid surgery, but now most causes are **idiopathic**. Voice is preserved, with stridor most evident on exertion. Flexible laryngoscopy reveals limitation of abduction of the cords on inspiration. Management includes observation only, a choice of intralaryngeal procedures to increase the airway at the glottic level, or tracheostomy.

Malignancy

Malignant lesions of the larynx and hypopharynx can present with stridor due to **tumour obstruction** of the airway or by causing **vocal cord palsy** and **oedema**. Stridor can also occur after radiation for laryngeal cancers. It is not always possible to secure the airway before tracheostomy. Debulking the tumour to improve the airway while awaiting definitive management is an option. For factors that determine treatment, see Chapter 19. Tumours presenting with stridor are usually well advanced locally and may need total laryngectomy for clearance (Fig. 12.7).

Intubation trauma

Intubation for any length of time causes laryngeal inflammation. Extensive inflammation and ulceration lead to **fibrosis** and **scarring.** This usually affects the subglottis. Neonates tolerate intubation for weeks with little long-term harm, but it is reasonable to consider conversion to tracheostomy after a week to 10 days of intubation in adults if no extubation is planned. Reconstruction of the stenotic segment is needed in established stenosis.

Laryngeal trauma

Blunt and **penetrating** trauma cause airway obstruction. Other findings include hoarseness, subcutaneous emphysema and haemoptysis. Intubation causes further disruption to the larynx and the airway is best secured by an urgent tracheostomy.

Angioedema

Angioedema is explained by abnormal vascular permeability beneath the dermis. The causes are shown in Box 12.4. The onset of oedema can occur within a few hours and can lead to rapid airway obstruction. Management is primarily medical with epinephrine, steroids and antihistamines.

Surgical management of the acutely obstructed airway

Children should be transferred to a centre with medical and nursing expertise in managing paediatric airway problems, where the airway is secured in conjunction with a direct laryngoscopy. If endotracheal intubation is difficult, a laryngeal mask airway or a rigid bronchoscope is used to maintain the airway and ventilate the patient while tracheostomy is performed. Tracheostomy in children, especially neonates, is associated with a high risk of complications. If rapid deterioration occurs and there is not sufficient time for a tracheostomy, a cricothyrotomy can provide emergency oxygenation. In adults, endotracheal intubation is usually possible. Adult patients with sup-

---

Box 12.4 **Causes of angioedema**

The following are possible causes:
- IgE mediated – atopy, allergens, physical stimuli;
- complement mediated – hereditary (production of low or dysfunctional C1 INH*);
- non-immunologic – drug induced (e.g. angiotensin-converting inhibitors, beta lactam antibiotics);
- idiopathic.
  * C1 INH: C1-esterase inhibitor.

raglottitis may be observed in a high dependency setting. Obstructive lesions may need tracheostomy or debulking.

Tracheostomy

Tracheostomy can be used for three reasons: to bypass the upper airway in airway obstruction, to provide pulmonary toilet and for access during head and neck surgery. This is performed under general anaesthesia if possible.

Ideally, a horizontal incision is made 2 cm above the suprasternal notch. Dissection proceeds in the midline to separate the strap muscles and expose the thyroid isthmus, which is ligated and cut. The tracheal rings are exposed and 'stay' sutures inserted, especially in children. These help with finding the track should the tube become displaced after operation. A vertical slit tracheostomy is made through the third and fourth rings, and the chosen tracheostomy tube is inserted (Fig. 12.8). The integrity of the tube and the cuff must be checked in advance. The tube is secured in place with sutures and tape as necessary. A tube change is performed after 4 to 7 days, allowing time for the track to mature. An uncuffed tube can be used at this time if there is little concern about significant aspiration. The cricoid cartilage must not be damaged to avoid stenosis.

Tracheostomy tubes

There are many types of tracheostomy tube, made of PVC, silicone or silver. A cuffed tube is usually used in the early days after operation, especially in a ventilated patient. This is changed to an uncuffed tube prior to discharge, unless there are significant problems with aspiration. This is often seen in patients with neurological disabili-

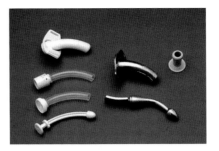

Figure 12.9 Tracheostomy tubes.

ties. A fenestrated tube with holes on the shoulder allows phonation when the tube is occluded. Most tracheostomy tubes used in hospital and community practice have an inner tube protruding just beyond the outer tube at its distal tip. The longer end of the inner tube picks up the dried mucus and can be removed for cleaning, while the outer tube is left in place (Fig. 12.9).

Care of a tracheostomy in the community

Patients who have a tracheostomy for chronic airway obstruction or pulmonary toilet may be managed at home. Care in the community needs skilled nursing. A good network of communication needs to be set up before discharge to ensure that the home is equipped with suction apparatus, a humidification system, if required, and a supply of spare tracheostomy tubes. The patient's family should be taught about tracheostomy care: how to perform competent suction and to replace the tube in the event of a blockage. A community physiotherapist and speech and language therapist may also be needed. Some problems faced in the community, such as narrowing of the tract and persistent granulations with bleeding around the stoma, may need specialist ENT advice.

Further reading

Leung AK, Cho H. (1999) Diagnosis of stridor in children. *American Family Physician*; **60**(8): 2289–96.

Lewarski JS. (2005) Long-term car of the patient with a tracheosotomy. *Respiratory Care*; **50**; (4): 534–7.

Mount J, Uner A, Kaku S. (2004) Pediatric wheezing and stridor. *Emergency Medical Services*; **33**(7): 55–56, 58–60.

Oberwaldner B, Eber E. (2006) Tracheostomy care in the home. *Paediatric Respiratory Review* **7**; (3): 185–90.

Yellon RF, Goldberg H. (2001) Update on gastroesophageal reflux disease in pediatric airway disorders. *American Journal of Medicine*; **111**(Suppl 8A): 78S–84S.

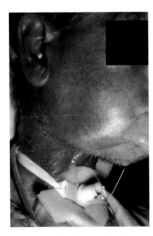

Figure 12.8 Total laryngectomy showing end tracheostoma with speaking valve in place.

CHAPTER 13

Swallowing Problems

Vinidh Paleri, Patrick J Bradley

OVERVIEW

- Dysphagia is the symptom of swallowing impairment.
- Swallowing can be divided into four stages: oral preparatory, oral, pharyngeal and oesophageal (Box 13.1).
- The majority of the swallowing mechanism is located above the clavicle.
- Weight loss is associated with significant disease or condition, difficult to reverse, and is usually a late sign.
- Aspiration is defined as liquid or solids penetrating below the level of the vocal cord and frequently may not precipitate any symptoms, coughing as a symptom is not reliable.
- Evaluation of the swallowing mechanism should be undertaken by a multidisciplinary team, not only for diagnosis but for treatment and rehabilitation.

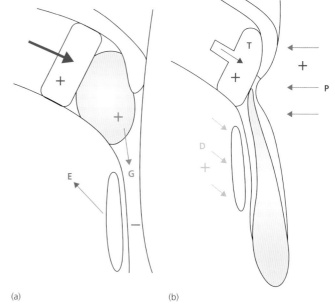

(a) (b)

Figure 13.1 (a) Pharyngeal phase of swallowing – early phase. (b) Pharyngeal phase of swallowing – late phase. D, depression; E, elevation; G, gravity; T, tongue; +, positive pressure; –, negative pressure.

Swallowing and its mechanisms

The pharyngeal stage is controlled at brain stem level (Fig. 13.1). The soft palate closes against the nasopharynx to prevent nasal regurgitation and laryngeal closure occurs to prevent aspiration. The epiglottis may play a greater role in directing the bolus into the piriform sinuses than in protecting the airway. Following laryngeal closure by cord adduction, the pharyngeal constrictor muscles sequentially contract to propel the bolus. The suprahyoid muscles raise the larynx, clearing the bolus down as the cricopharyngeal sphincter opens, admitting it to the upper oesophagus. The cricopharyngeus relaxes with laryngeal elevation, which mechanically pulls open the sphincter under bolus pressure. The oesophageal stage then follows for 8–20 seconds.

Symptoms

Swallowing problems present as difficulty in initiating the swallow, choking or coughing upon swallowing (aspiration) or a sensation

of obstruction in the neck or behind the sternum. Dysphagia may involve liquids, solids or both. Progressive difficulty with weight loss suggests malignant disease. Slow progression over years occurs in achalasia of the cardia and pharyngeal pouches (Zenker's diverticulum), associated with regurgitation of undigested food. Dry mouth (xerostomia), caused by autoimmune diseases (Sjogren's syndrome) and radiation therapy, also causes dysphagia (Box 13.2).

Box 13.1 **Stages of swallowing**

The four stages are:
- oral preparatory;
- oral;
- pharyngeal;
- oesophageal.

Box 13.2 **Investigations for dysphagia**

Primary care:
- full blood count;
- contrast swallow.

Secondary care:
- flexible and rigid endoscopy;
- videofluoroscopy;
- flexible endoscopic evaluation of swallowing;
- oesophageal manometry.

Weakness of the oral and lingual musculature leads to drooling and poor mastication. Altered sensation of the pharynx arising centrally in neurological disease, or peripherally after radiotherapy, delays initiation of the pharyngeal stage. This may cause aspiration, with coughing and choking, or a 'wet' voice quality. Aspiration also arises from laryngeal protective mechanism impairment in neurological or neoplastic processes. Aspiration can also be silent if laryngeal sensation is impaired, with risks of chest infection.

Clinical evaluation

There are good pointers towards the diagnosis in 80% of histories. Acute dysphagia is most usually caused by the presence of a foreign body or of a candidal infection. Dysphagia lasting longer than three weeks needs specialist referral. Otolaryngological examination must include flexible fibreoptic assessment of the pharynx (Fig. 13.2) and larynx. Lesions in the apex of the piriform sinus and the postcricoid region are not always apparent on flexible endoscopy and rigid endoscopy must be used when suspicion is high. Contrast swallows are useful to identify the presence and size of pharyngeal pouches, and oesophageal lesions. Videofluoroscopy provides dynamic assessment of the anatomy and coordination of the oral, pharyngeal and oesophageal stages of swallowing. The flow chart in Fig. 13.3 shows the role of investigations.

Common otolaryngological conditions causing chronic dysphagia are shown in Fig. 13.4.

Presbyphagia

Physiological changes occur in the swallowing reflex with ageing. There is reduction in muscle mass and strength. Presentation is that of chronic dysphagia with malnutrition and aspiration. Treatment involves modifying the consistency of food, and swallowing therapy with correction of concurrent contributory factors.

Globus pharyngeus

This is a sensation of a lump or tightness and irritation in the throat, where no organic cause is identified. It may be an atypical manifestation of gastro-oesophageal reflux or oesophageal dysmotility, or of psychogenic origin. Presentation is usually in middle age. Diagnosis is based on the history and lack of findings with no weight loss. Intermittent symptoms are typically between meals, accompanied by a continual urge to swallow. Unless presentation is atypical, further investigation is unwarranted. Treatment involves reassurance and an explanation, with anti-reflux therapy. Symptoms can last for up to 2 years and are often recurrent.

Pharyngeal pouch (Zenker's diverticulum)

There is natural weakness in the posterior aspect of the hypopharynx (Fig. 13.5), between the fibres of the thyropharyngeus and the cricopharyngeus muscles (upper oesophageal sphincter) of the inferior pharyngeal constrictor. Pulsion diverticula can form at this site. Various hypotheses of aetiology include poor relaxation of the cricopharyngeal muscle during swallowing, increased resting tone of the muscle and myopathy of the cricopharyngeus.

The condition usually arises in the elderly, and presents with progressive dysphagia and weight loss. Symptoms include regurgitation of undigested food many hours after eating, gurgling sounds in the neck during swallowing, halitosis, coughing episodes and aspiration. Endoscopic examination may reveal some pooling of residue in the hypopharynx, and reflux. Contrast swallow establishes the diagnosis (Fig. 13.6). Patients are prone to oesophageal perforation during endoscopic examination if a pouch is not recognized pre-operatively. Treatment depends on the size of the pouch and its symptoms. Small pouches discovered incidentally need no treatment. The management of larger, symptomatic pouches includes endoscopic stapling of the party wall between the pouch and the oesophagus to prevent food from stagnating in the pouch (Fig. 13.7). There is a very small incidence of malignancy in these pouches and careful telescopic inspection is essential prior to stapling. Difficult exposure due to a short neck and an anteriorly placed larynx may preclude stapling. An external excision of the pouch is then needed.

Postcricoid web

This condition is usually found in women in their forties and fifties, in association with iron deficiency anaemia and weight loss. The onset is gradual and patients have altered dietary habits to compensate for the dysphagia. Examination findings may include angular cheilitis and atrophy of the dorsum of the tongue from iron deficiency (Fig. 13.8). Contrast X-ray shows a thin filling defect, usually arising on the anterior wall. Early webs may be reversed by iron supplementation, but the majority need rigid endoscopic dilatation of the web for relief. A postcricoid carcinoma, unlike other hypopharyngeal cancer, is more commonly found in younger women, and up to two-thirds have experienced the presence of previous or persistent symptoms of a web.

Neurological diseases

Myasthenia gravis, multiple sclerosis, motor neurone disease, muscular dystrophies and other degenerative disorders may affect swallowing. The problem is with initiation of swallow for both solids and liquids, and symptoms are usually progressive. Swallowing therapy may be helpful. These patients are prone to aspiration due to diminished sensation of the pharynx and impaired lingual and pharyngeal constrictor activity. If aspiration is intractable, and the patient is having difficulty maintaining daily calorific intake, tube feeding (by gastrostomy) may be considered.

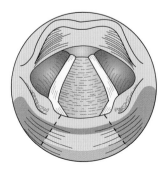

Figure 13.2 Regions of the hypopharynx (purple – piriform sinus, blue – postcricoid space, green – posterior pharyngeal wall).

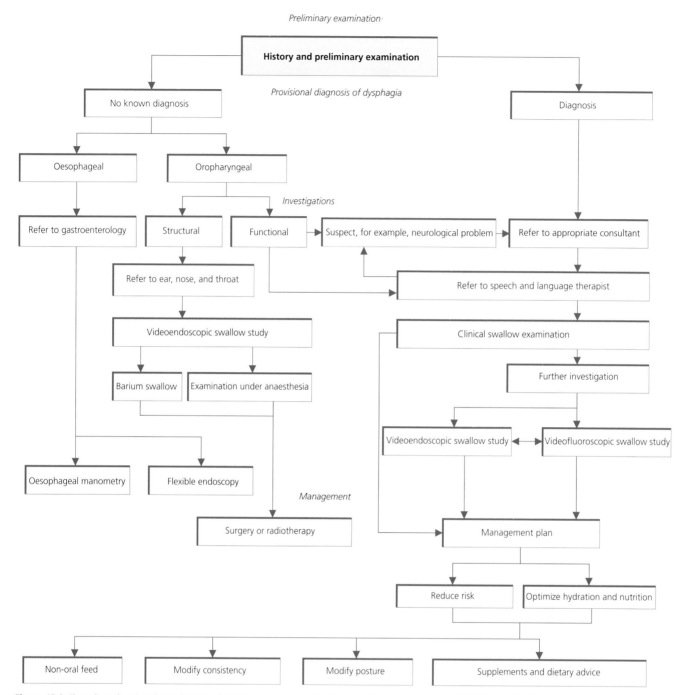

Figure 13.3 Flow chart showing the evaluation of dysphagia. Reproduced with permission from Leslie *et al.* (2003) *British Medical Journal*; **326**: 433–6.

Acute onset palsy of the vagus presents with dysphagia, aspiration (Fig. 13.9) and a breathy voice. The aetiology is often idiopathic. Possible causes are viral neuritis or damage to the neural microvasculature by underlying systemic causes such as diabetes mellitus. Structural lesions must be excluded by imaging the course of the recurrent laryngeal nerve from the skull base to the diaphragm for left cord palsy, and to the superior mediastinum for right cord palsy. Improvement in symptoms may take place by compensation from the contralateral cord over a few months. A head turn to the affected side on swallowing can help to reduce aspiration. If aspiration continues with poor speech, the affected cord can be moved surgically to meet its fellow, reducing aspiration and improving the voice.

Percutaneous gastrostomy

High-dose radiation therapy to a primary site of cancer-related dysphagia, especially when combined with concurrent chemotherapy, leads to severe mucositis and restriction in oral intake. Supplementation of feeds may be needed by nasogastric tube or preferably a gastrostomy. A gastrostomy tube is inserted before treatment under endoscopic, ultrasound or fluoroscopic guidance without the need for laparotomy (Fig. 13.10). It is easily performed with minimal morbidity. It is also widely used in neurological practice, when long-term dysphagia is expected, being more comfortable than a nasogastric tube and offering the patient greater mobility.

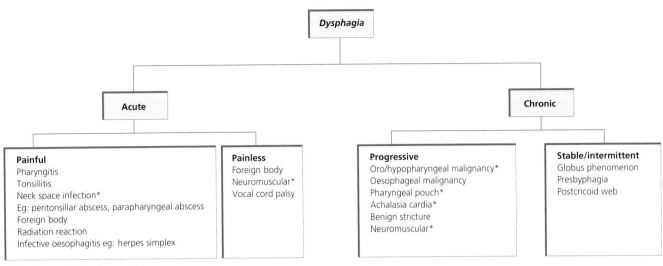

Figure 13.4 Flow chart showing the differential diagnostic options for dysphagia of otolaryngological origin.

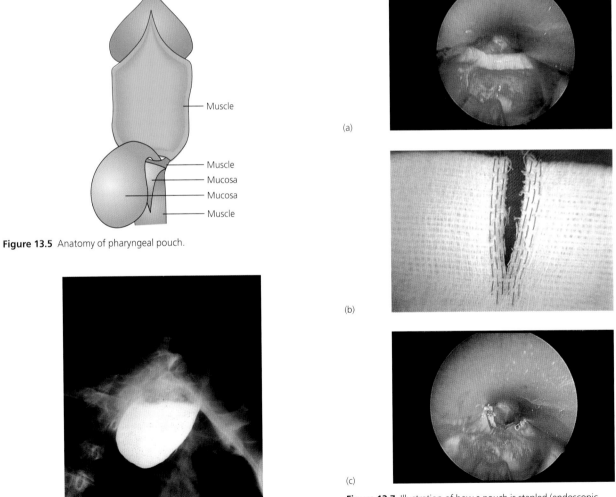

Figure 13.5 Anatomy of pharyngeal pouch.

Figure 13.6 Radiological image of a 'large pharyngeal pouch'.

Figure 13.7 Illustration of how a pouch is stapled (endoscopic cricopharyngeal myotomy): (a) a prominent cricopharyngeal 'bar' muscle, the oesophagus opening anteriorly and the pouch posteriorly; (b) the method of stapling, with two parallel rows of three sets of staples, between which the muscle and the mucosa are divided; (c) the bar has been divided – increasing the opening into the oesophagus.

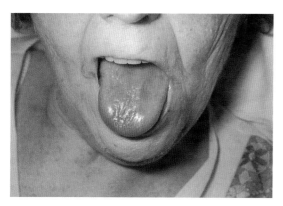

Figure 13.8 Angular chelitis and atrophic glossitis.

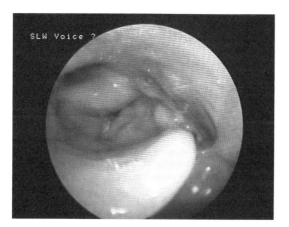

Figure 13.9 Residual coloured contrast remaining in the hypopharynx.

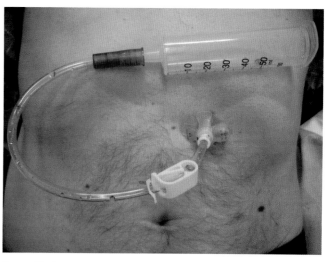

Figure 13.10 A percutaneous gastrostomy.

gies to improve nutritional status and prevent chest infections or pneumonia. Common interventions may include head or body postures to improve control and direction of bolus flow, manoeuvres to improve airway closure and protection or the efficiency of bolus clearance, exercises to increase the range or strength of movements of the swallowing musculature and/or dietary modifications to suit the patient's abilities.

Swallowing therapy

Speech and language therapists may be involved in the management of patients with oropharyngeal dysphagia. Following clinical assessment, and videofluoroscopy or endoscopic assessment when indicated, they may recommend management or rehabilitation strate-

Further reading

Amin MR, Postma GN. (2004) Office evaluation of swallowing. *Ear, Nose & Throat Journal*; **83**(7,Suppl 2): 13–16.

Hiss, SG, Postma, GN. (2003) Fiberoptic endoscopic evaluation of swallowing. *Laryngoscope*; **113**(8): 1386–93.

Leslie P, Carding PN, Wilson JA. (2003) Investigation and management of chronic dysphagia. *British Medical Journal*; **326**: 433–6.

Spieker MR. (2000) Evaluating dysphagia. *American Family Physician*; **61**: 3639–48.

CHAPTER 14

Snoring and Obstructive Sleep Apnoea

Anshul Sama

OVERVIEW

- Snoring, noisy breathing during sleep, is caused by vibration of one or more areas of the upper airway.
- Such noisy breathing occurs in 45% of the population from time to time and an estimated 25% are habitual snorers.
- Although snoring is the cardinal symptom of obstructive sleep apnoea, the prevalence of obstructive sleep apnoea is notably lower at 0.5–4%.

Spectrum of the condition

Snoring and obstructive sleep apnoea form the opposite ends of a spectrum of disorders under the umbrella of obstructive sleep-related breathing disorders (SRBDs) (Fig. 14.1). Depending on the degree of obstruction and associated symptoms, individuals are categorized into one of the following categories.

Simple snoring is disruptive snoring without any impact on the patient's sleep pattern or increased daytime sleepiness. As the obstruction increases, greater respiratory effort leads to increased sleep disruption and daytime sleepiness. **Upper airways resistance syndrome (UARS)** is categorized by the presence of these symptoms without evidence of obstructive apnoea or oxygen desaturation.

There is increased respiratory effort recognized by oesophageal pressure analysis. Further progression of airway obstruction leads to near total or total obstruction of airflow. **Obstructive sleep apnoea hypopnoea syndrome (OSAHS)** comprises excessive daytime sleepiness with interrupted and repeated collapse of the upper airway during sleep, causing oxygen desaturation. Collapse may be complete with cessation of airflow (apnoea), or partial with significant hypoventilation (hypopnoea).

The frequency of apnoea and hypopnoea is used to grade the severity of OSAHS as the apnoea/hypopnoea index (AHI), or the respiratory disturbance index (RDI). OSAHS is mild (5–14 events per hour), moderate (15–30 events per hour) or severe (more than 30 events per hour). Clinically significant OSAHS is only likely to be present when the AHI is greater than 15 events per hour, in association with unexplained daytime sleepiness or a minimum of two of the other features of the condition identified in Box 14.1.

Aetiology

Snoring and obstructive apnoea only occur during sleep. In humans, the airway between the posterior end of the nose and the larynx is unprotected by cartilaginous or bony structures and is reliant on muscle tone for its patency. With the onset of sleep, pharyngeal muscle tone falls progressively as sleep deepens. This phenomenon is present in all

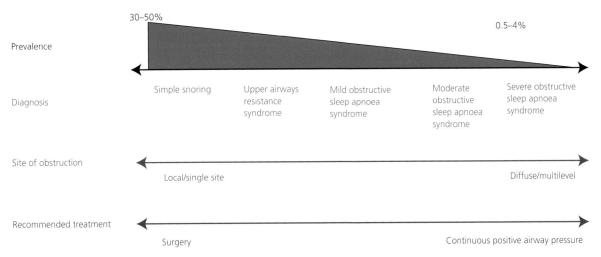

Figure 14.1 Sleep-related breathing disorders – a spectrum of conditions.

humans and yet not all snore or have OSAHS. Factors that have been found to increase the risk of SRBDs are as follows.

- **Age.** There is a progressive increase in the prevalence of snoring and obstructive sleep apnoea up to the sixth and seventh decades of life independent of the body mass index (BMI).
- **Sex.** Men have between a two- and fivefold increased risk of OSAHS compared with age- and weight-matched women. The reasons for the sex difference are unknown. The prevalence of snoring and obstructive sleep apnoea in women increases post-menopause. Oestrogen plus progesterone replacement therapy in post-menopausal women has been shown to reduce occurrences.
- **Obesity.** The most important risk factor. The prevalence of respiratory events (RDI) has been shown to directly correlate with BMI. Seventy per cent of individuals with BMI of 40 or greater suffer with OSAHS. Conversely, up to 50% of patients with OSAHS may have a BMI below 30. Central obesity indicators such as neck circumference index and waist to hip ratio are better predictors of OSAHS than obesity or BMI in general.
- **Obstructive upper airway anatomy.** Craniofacial abnormalities are associated with a higher prevalence of SRBDs. These include abnormalities such as retro- or micrognathia, midfacial or mandibular hypoplasia and macroglossia. Adenotonsillar hypertrophy is common in children as a cause of snoring and OSAHS. Obstruction of the nasal airway due to turbinate hypertrophy, septal deviations or nasal polyposis increases upper airway resistance. These contribute to snoring and UARS, but are unlikely to be the sole cause for OSAHS.
- **Social habits.** Smoking and alcohol consumption increase the risk of SRBDs.
- **Other risk factors.** The relative risk of OSAHS may be two- to fourfold greater in first degree relatives even after adjustment for BMI and craniofacial variations. Certain medical conditions such as hypothyroidism and acromegaly are associated with OSAHS. Neuromuscular diseases also predispose to OSAHS, although central apnoeas are more likely. Drugs associated with central depression such as hypnotics and opioids increase the risk of SRBDs. Chronic lung disease does not pose a direct risk for SRBDs. However, in both obstructive and restricted lung disease, OSAHS tends to be more severe with deeper events of oxygen desaturation resulting from hypoventilation and the lower lung reserve.

Consequences of sleep-related breathing disorders

Although simple snoring has a significant social impact, it has no detrimental impact on an individual's health. However, OSAHS is known to have important cardiovascular and other consequences.

Neurocognitive effects

Excessive daytime sleepiness (EDS) is the commonest complaint of patients with obstructive sleep apnoea. Cognitive performance is notably impaired with deterioration in memory, intellectual capacity and motor co-ordination. There is an increase in accident rates amongst patients with OSAHS. Sleepiness at the wheel is estimated to cause 20% of road traffic accidents on major highways.

Cardiovascular consequences

There is compelling evidence that OSAHS is associated and contributes to systemic hypertension. This association is independent of confounding factors such as obesity, age, gender and alcohol consumption. Furthermore, treatment with continuous positive airway pressure (CPAP) reduces blood pressure by up to 5 mmHg over 24 hours. There are some data suggesting an association between OSAHS and coronary artery disease and cerebrovascular events.

Other issues

Patients with OSAHS have been known to have potential problems with impotence and increased likelihood of gastro-oesophageal reflux.

Assessment

The aims are to:
1 identify if the patient has OSAHS;
2 identify the potential causes and predisposing factors;
3 localize the level(s) of obstruction in the upper airway.

The Epworth sleepiness scale (ESS) is a validated method of identifying EDS. However, the correlation between ESS and OSAHS is relatively weak and it cannot be used as a screening tool for OSAHS. Physical examination of the upper airway is essential and is usually performed by an ENT surgeon. However, there is poor correlation between the clinical findings and predictability of OSAHS. A formal assessment of nasal airway and pharyngeal anatomy needs to be undertaken, preferably with an endoscope (flexible or rigid). An assessment should be made of the oropharyngeal inlet including tonsil, tongue and mandibular size. The possibility of hyperthyroidism, acromegaly and Marfan's syndrome should always be considered in patients presenting with snoring or OSAHS.

Sleep studies

Sleep studies are indicated in all patients presenting with snoring or suspected sleep apnoea. OSAHS should always be excluded in patients before considering surgery for snoring. OSAHS can be present in over 30% of snorers presenting without symptoms of overt sleepiness. Patients with chronic obstructive pulmonary disease (COPD) and snoring should have an urgent sleep study as the combination is potentially dangerous. All patients who drive long distances and/or heavy goods vehicles, or handle hazardous machinery as part of their profession, must have a sleep study as part of their assessment. There are many levels of sleep study depending on the local circumstances.

Polysomnography

Polysomnography (PSG) is the gold standard for diagnosis of OSAHS. The technique entails an inpatient study involving overnight assessment of a number of measures, including: EEG, electromyogram, electro-oculogram, respiratory airflow, thoraco-abdominal movement, ECG, oximetry, body position, snoring sound and video. Clearly, it is a relatively intrusive and costly study whose interpretation can be complex (Fig. 14.2).

Treatment options

The choice of treatment is dictated by the following.
- **Diagnosis.** In moderate to severe OSAHS, the aim is to eliminate the episodes of apnoeas/hypopnoeas, desaturations and associated daytime sleepiness. The ideal treatment is CPAP. In the simple snorer, the aim is a reduction of the duration and intensity of snoring to socially acceptable levels. Lifestyle changes, oral devices and limited surgery are appropriate. In UARS and mild OSAHS, the aim is reduction in snoring but also the upper airway resistance with sleep fragmentation. Most modalities of treatment are appropriate depending on patient choice and the predominant symptom – snoring noise reduction or sleep disturbance.
- **Accurate localization of the level of airway obstruction.** Other than lifestyle changes and CPAP, other modalities of treatment are

site specific. Therefore, the efficacy of the treatment is dependent on accurate localization of the obstruction. Clinical and radiological examinations are poor for localizing the level of obstruction. Fibreoptic upper airway endoscopy, with or without sedation, is of limited use, as it is not performed during natural sleep and is unipositional. Upper airway pressure recordings and acoustic reflectometry are promising techniques, although they are not widely available or practised in the UK.

Behavioural changes

For simple snoring, simple measures, such as allowing the partner to fall asleep first, using ear plugs, or sleeping on one side rather than the back, can often suffice.

Weight loss

Obesity is the single most important factor in increasing upper airway resistance. Weight reduction has been shown to reduce snoring and the number of apnoeas and hypopnoeas, and improve sleep efficiency and oxygenation. The most dramatic results have been reported with surgical weight loss. It should be recognized that substantial weight loss by non-surgical means is both difficult to achieve and hard to maintain.

Lifestyle changes

Patients should be encouraged to stop smoking. Although there is evidence linking smoking with OSAHS, there is no evidence that stopping smoking improves apnoeic events. Alcohol, especially close to bedtime, exaggerates loss of pharyngeal muscle tone during sleep and episodes of airway collapse. For similar reasons, sleeping tablets, sedative antihistamines and tranquillizers should be avoided at bedtime.

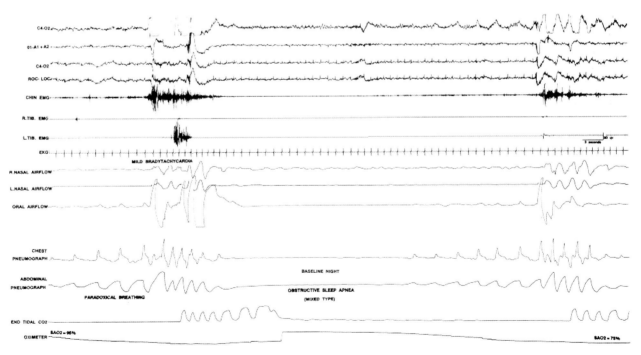

Figure 14.2 Polysomnography trace.

Continuous positive airway pressure

CPAP applied via a nasal mask has been shown to be the most effective treatment for OSAHS. It may eliminate apnoeas/hypopnoeas and improve daytime alertness, neurocognitive functions, mood and cardiovascular sequelae. Unfortunately, it suffers from compliance limitations. One-third of patients offered CPAP are unwilling to use it and nocturnal use averages only 4–5 hours per night. Compliance can be improved by initial habituation to the mask for several days before CPAP usage, eliminating oral leakage with chin straps and heated humidification to reduce nasal dryness, Bi-level positive airway pressure (BIPAP) or Auto-CPAP to reduce exhalation pressure. The most important factor is supportive and accessible medical staff.

Intra-oral appliance

Several intra-oral devices have been designed to enlarge the pharyngeal airway by moving and fixing the mandible in an anterior position. These are effective in improving snoring and mild OSAHS. Side effects relating to excessive salivation, jaw discomfort, teeth/gum discomfort and temporomandibular joint dysfunction affect the majority of patients.

Pharmacological treatment

Drugs used in the treatment of OSAHS are either respiratory stimulants for increasing upper airway muscle tone, or drugs for treating excessive daytime hypersomnolence. Protryptyline, acetazolamide and progesterone are respiratory stimulants and suppress rapid eye movement sleep (when airway collapse is most likely). These drugs are not curative in the treatment of OSAHS. There is some evidence to show that the addition of alerting drugs, such as modafinil, may be beneficial in reducing daytime sleepiness in those who remain sleepy despite CPAP usage.

Upper airway surgery

The success of upper airway surgery depends on accurate identification of the level/s of obstruction, and effective surgical treatment. Identification of the level of obstruction has traditionally been based on clinical assessment and/or investigations under sedation.

Tracheostomy was the first surgical procedure used in the treatment of OSAHS. It is rarely performed today. Current surgical approaches are designed to widen the upper airway: nasal, oropharyngeal or retrolingual. These procedures are usually single site and non-invasive for simple snoring, and multiple level and invasive for moderate to severe OSAHS.

Nasal surgery

Nasal disease increases the upper airway resistance, with increased negative pressure in the pharynx during inspiration. Surgical correction of a deviated septum, removal of nasal polyps and turbinate reduction can reduce upper airway resistance. However, the reported impact on snoring is variable (39–87%) and there is relapse after several years. In patients with OSAHS, nasal procedures can improve compliance with nasal CPAP but they do not improve OSAHS *per se*.

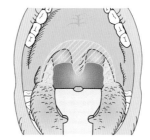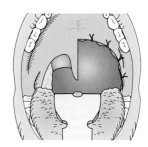

Figure 14.3 Traditional uvulopalatopharyngoplasty (UPPP).

Uvulopalatopharyngoplasty

Uvulopalatopharyngoplasty (UPPP) has a long track record for widening the oropharyngeal airway. The procedure involves tonsillectomy, uvulectomy and excision of a variable segment of the soft palate (Fig. 14.3). In the appropriately selected group, i.e. suspected obstruction solely at the level of the soft palate/oropharynx, success rates for simple snoring vary between 75 and 85% and around 50% for OSAHS. It is notable that the success rate decreases with increasing follow-up periods.

Laser-assisted uvulopalatoplasty

Laser-assisted uvulopalatoplasty (LAUP), although originally developed as a modification of the traditional UPPP, has evolved notably in the last decade. There are many techniques in the literature.

Radiofrequency

Radiofrequency (RF) procedures of the tonsil, palate and tongue base are based on the principle of submucosal application of low-frequency radiowaves to create thermic lesions and subsequent volume reduction and scarring (Figs 14.4 and 14.5).

Maxillofacial and multilevel surgery

Maxillofacial and multilevel surgery is usually performed for patients with moderate to severe OSAHS. It includes a range of procedures to improve the retrolingual airway and the retropalatal airway. These are extremely invasive and their use is limited to patients who fail to use CPAP.

Snoring and obstructive sleep apnoea in children

Although OSAHS in children has many similarities with the adult form, there are some notable differences (Table 14.1). Unlike adults, the incidence is equal in both sexes and does not increase with age. The peak occurrence is between the ages of 2 and 5 years, when the adenoids and tonsils are largest in relation to the oropharyngeal size. Children with OSAHS frequently show signs of failure to thrive rather than obesity. Symptoms in children are similar to those in adults, with the exception of sleepiness. Paradoxically, children often demonstrate restlessness and hyperactivity. Other potential consequences in children include secondary enuresis.

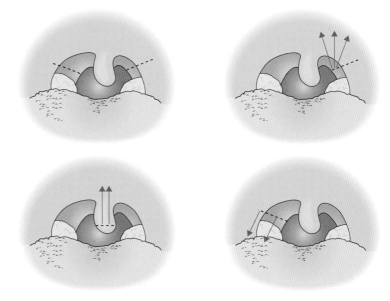

Figure 14.4 Minimally invasive radiofrequency techniques (cautery-assisted uvulopalatoplasty; CAUP).

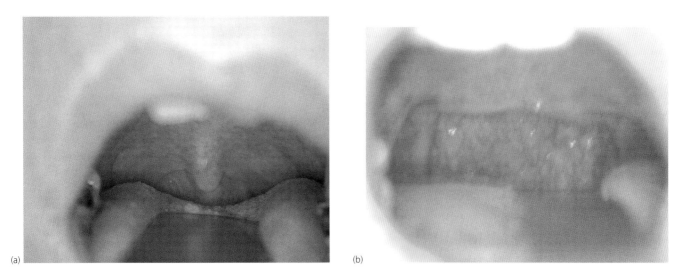

(a)

(b)

Figure 14.5 Outcome with (cautery-assisted uvulopalatoplasty; CAUP) palatal surgery. (a) Before. (b) After.

Table 14.1 Differences in characteristics of obstructive sleep apnoea between children and adults

	Children	Adults
Age	Peak: 2–5 years	Increases with age
Gender	Male = female	Male > female
Weight	Usually undernourished	Usually obese
Daytime somnolence	Uncommon	Primary symptom
Neurobehaviour	Hyperactive, developmental delay	Cognitive impairment, impaired vigilance

Although OSAHS in children is associated with adenotonsillar hypertrophy (Fig. 14.6), it is unlikely to be the only cause. Other anatomical factors that are predisposing to OSAHS include choanal stenosis/atresia, macroglossia, micrognathia, midface hypoplasia (e.g. Down's, Crouzon's and Apert's syndromes, achondroplasia) and mandibular hypoplasia (e.g. Pierre-Robin and Cornelle De Lange syndrome).

Medical sequelae, such as pulmonary hypertension, systemic hypertension, cor pulmonale and congestive heart failure, are rare. Neurobehavioural and developmental consequences are more com-

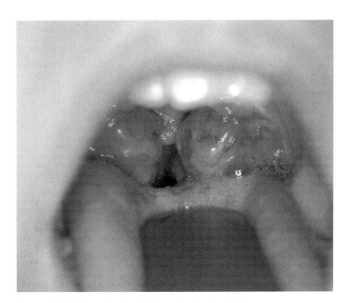

Figure 14.6 Obstructive tonsillar hypertrophy in a child.

mon, including poor school performance, poor learning skills, attention deficit hyperactivity disorder and behavioural problems.

Key points

- SRBDs include a spectrum of conditions from simple snoring to severe obstructive sleep apnoea.
- OSAHS is associated with systemic hypertension and notable neurocognitive sequelae.
- Patients who must be considered for sleep studies are:
  - those with COPD as the combination is potentially dangerous;
  - those describing daytime sleepiness and those who work with dangerous machinery or drive for their profession;
  - those being considered for surgery for snoring.
- Surgical procedures for SRBD should be guided by the diagnosis and level/s of obstruction.
- There are notable differences between the adult and childhood forms of OSAHS.

Further reading

Faber CE, Grymer L. (2003) Available techniques for objective assessment of upper airway narrowing in snoring and sleep apnoea. *Sleep and Breathing*; **7**: 77–87.

Friedman M, Tanyeri H, Lim JW *et al.* (2000) Effect of improved nasal breathing on obstructive sleep apnea. *Otolaryngolology – Head and Neck Surgery*; **122**: 71–4.

Gozal D. (1998) Sleep disordered breathing and school performance in children. *Pediatrics*; **102**: 616–20.

Hicklin LA, Tostevin P, Dasan S. (2000) Retrospective survey of long-term results and patient satisfaction with uvulopalatopharyngoplasty for snoring. *Journal of Laryngology and Otolaryngology*; **114**: 675–81.

Marcus CL. (2001) Sleep disordered breathing in children. *American Journal of Respiratory Critical Care Medicine*; **164**: 16–30.

Miljeteig H, Mateika S, Haight JS, Cole P, Hoffstein V. (1994) Subjective and objective assessment of uvulopalatopharyngoplasty for treatment of snoring and obstructive sleep apnea. *American Journal of Respiratory Critical Care Medicine*; **150**: 1286–90.

Ross SD, Allen IE, Harrison KJ *et al.* (1999) *Systematic review of the literature regarding the diagnosis of sleep apnea.* Agency for Health Care Policy and Research, Rockville, MD. AHCPR publication No. 99-E002, www.ncbi.nlm.nih.gov/books/bv.fcgi?rid=hstat1.chapter.2 [accessed on 28 April 2003].

Worsnop CJ, Naughton MT, Barter CE *et al.* (1998) The prevalence of obstructive sleep apnoea in hypertensives. *American Journal of Respiratory Critical Care Medicine*; **157**: 111–15.

CHAPTER 15

Hoarseness and Voice Problems

Julian McGlashan, Declan Costello, Patrick J Bradley

OVERVIEW

- Hoarseness or dysphonia is a symptom of altered laryngeal function and merits investigation and treatment.
- The causes of hoarseness include; structural and neoplastic, inflammatory, neuromuscular and muscle tension imbalance, and most patients have a combination of causes.
- Patients who smoke and are hoarse only, inspection of the larynx will always identify the cause, a chest x-ray is indicated when patients have additional symptoms – dyspnoea, chest pain or haemoptysis.
- Voice disorders should be investigated and managed by a multidisciplinary team and may require many tests including stroboscopy and voice analysis.

Box 15.2 **Commonest voice complaints**

- Change in voice quality (hoarseness, roughness and breathiness)
- A deeper or higher pitched voice that is not appropriate for the age and gender
- Problems controlling the voice, described as pitch breaks, squeaky voice or the voice cutting out
- Difficulty making oneself heard in a noisy environment or in raising the voice
- Efforts in producing voice
- Reduced stamina of voice, which tires with use
- Difficulties or restrictions in the use of voice at different times of the day or related to specific daily, social or occupationally-related tasks
- Reduced ability to communicate effectively
- Difficulty in singing
- Throat-related symptoms (soreness, discomfort, aching, dryness, mucus) particularly related to voice use
- Emotional and psychological aspects of the above

The need to use the voice (Box 15.1) for prolonged periods, especially at raised intensity levels, increases the risk of dysphonia. The commonest voice complaints are outlined in Box 15.2.

Anatomy, physiology and pathophysiology

The vocal cords are attached anteriorly to the thyroid cartilage and posteriorly to a pair of arytenoid cartilages, perched on the superior rim of the cricoid cartilage. The intrinsic laryngeal muscles abduct the cords for respiration and adduct the cords for lower airway protection, coughing and phonation (Fig. 15.1). The vocal cords are folds of mucosa and are better called vocal folds. They consist of a superficial epithelial layer separated from the underlying ligament and muscle by the so-called Reinke's space. This allows the epithelial layer to slide and oscillate passively over the ligament (Fig. 15.2). The larynx is divided into three regions: supraglottis, glottis and subglottis (Fig. 15.3).

Box 15.1 **Definition of a normal voice**

A pragmatic definition of a **normal voice** is one that is:
- audible in a wide range of acoustic settings;
- appropriate for the gender and age of speaker;
- capable of fulfilling its linguistic and paralinguistic functions;
- not easily fatigued;
- not associated with phonatory discomfort or pain.

Aetiology of voice problems

Voice problems are classified as: structural/neoplastic, inflammatory, neuromuscular and muscle tension imbalance. Many patients have evidence of more than one. A vocal fold polyp (Fig. 15.4), for instance (structural/neoplastic cause), may arise as a result of primary muscle tension from voice abuse, such as shouting, during viral upper respiratory tract infection (inflammation). This polyp can cause secondary trauma to the vocal folds (inflammation) and muscle tension imbalance. An important part of the assessment of a patient is the determination of which of these conditions are present, which are primary and which are secondary, and which cause the complaint.

Guidelines and referral

Examination of the larynx is rarely possible by the general practitioner. As laryngeal visualization is the key examination, most patients need to be referred. Patients with persistent hoarseness or change in voice for 3 weeks, especially smokers and heavy drinkers aged 40 years or older, need urgent chest X-rays to exclude recurrent laryngeal nerve palsy from lung cancer, and referral to an ENT surgeon. Positive X-ray findings indicate urgent referral to a lung cancer specialist team. Negative X-ray findings with upper aerodi-

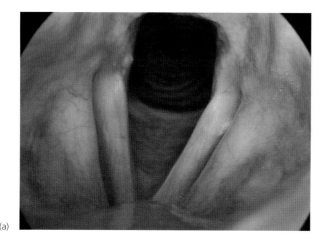

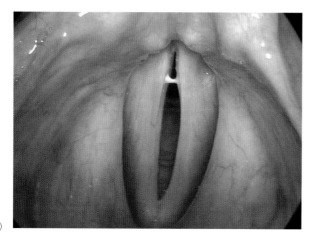

Figure 15.1 Vocal folds in abduction for respiration (a) and adduction for phonation (b).

gestive tract symptoms (Table 15.1) demand referral to a head and neck cancer specialist team. Others should be seen in a specialist voice disorders clinic.

Assessment

Comprehensive assessment of a voice problem includes the items listed in Box 15.3.

The first aim is to identify the presence of the main aetiological factors (Fig. 15.5). History details are outlined in Table 15.2. It is essential to decide whether the voice is rough, breathy, weak or strained, its appropriateness for the age and gender of the patient, whether the voice is too loud or too soft and whether vocal character is variable.

A flexible endoscope allows inspection of the vocal tract from nasal cavity to larynx. It is the preferred technique in neuromuscular and muscle tension imbalance disorders. A rigid endoscope placed on the tongue provides higher quality, with larger images, and is better for examining the vocal fold structure and function. The use of stroboscopic light improves the accuracy of diagnosis. Recording images digitally means that they can be stored, and recalled for slow motion playback (Fig. 15.6). Neck masses must be sought, and abnormalities of shape and movement of the laryngeal cartilages must be identi-

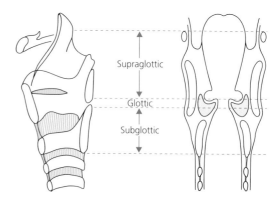

Figure 15.3 Sagittal and coronal views of the larynx showing regions.

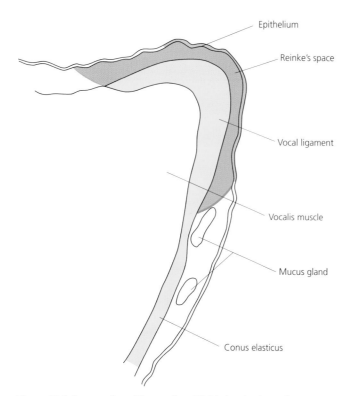

Figure 15.2 Cross-section of the vocal cord (fold) showing layered structure.

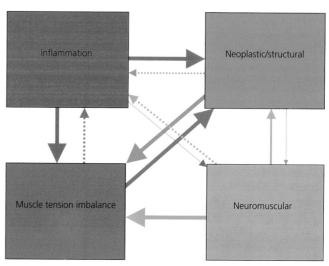

Figure 15.4 Example of structural abnormality: vocal polyp.

Table 15.1 Symptoms and signs of laryngeal and lung cancer

Laryngeal cancer (UK incidence of 3.7/100 000; Cancer Research UK)	Lung cancer (UK incidence of 63.9/100 000; Cancer Research UK)
• Hoarseness: • Rough voice due to vocal cord lesion • (A subtle change in voice may be only symptom) • Unexplained lump in neck recently appeared or changed over 3–6 weeks • Unexplained pain in head and neck region • Referred otalgia (normal otoscopy) • Unexplained persistent sore or painful throat • Other: • Inspiratory stridor • Haemoptysis • Dysphagia	• Haemoptysis or any of the following unexplained persistent (>3 weeks) symptoms and signs: • Hoarseness • Weak breathy voice due to vocal cord palsy • Cervical and/or supraclavicular lymphadenopathy • Dyspnoea • Chest and/or shoulder pain • Weight loss • Finger clubbing • Cough with or without any of the above • Features suggestive of metastases from lung cancer

fied. Tenderness of the extralaryngeal muscles may indicate increased muscle tension.

Electromyography is helpful in detecting paresis and in distinguishing cricoarytenoid joint fixation from vocal cord palsy. Microlaryngoscopy is helpful in cases of persistent chronic laryngitis or when outpatient laryngoscopy is not possible. Laryngopharyngeal reflux (Fig. 15.7) can be investigated by 24-hour pH measurements with probes coupled to oesophageal impedance measurements.

Treatment

Treatment options (Table 15.3) depend on the diagnosis, reasons for seeking referral, vocal requirements and risk/benefit of intervention. If the diagnosis is not initially clear, a trial of simple vocal hygiene measures, medical treatment or voice therapy can be tried. Primary surgery is performed for suspected neoplastic lesions,

Box 15.3 Requirements for comprehensive assessment of a voice problem

Requirements are:
- detailed clinical history;
- perceptual evaluation of the voice quality;
- flexible nasoendoscopic examination of vocal tract for (a) structure and (b) function;
- videolaryngostroboscopic assessment of vocal fold vibration;
- neck inspection and palpation for:
  - lymphadenopathy and other masses;
  - increased muscle tension and imbalance;
  - larynx position in neck and relationship of the thyroid and cricoid cartilages;
- neck, back and overall body posture;
- breathing patterns during speech;
- neurological assessment;
- psychological assessment.

Further investigations
- diagnostic microlaryngoscopy;
- quality of life measures using validated questionnaires;
- objective measurements of vocal function, e.g. acoustic, electrolaryngographic and aerodynamic measures, electromyography;
- 24-hour dual-site pH monitoring with impedance;
- oesophagogastroduodenoscopy.

leucoplakia (white mucosal lesions) and many cases of papillomas, polyps and vocal cord palsy (Fig. 15.8). Other structural lesions may require surgery. Post-operative voice therapy may also help.

Structural/neoplastic conditions

The voice depends on the effects of the lesion on vocal fold vibration and glottic closure. If the vocal fold vibration is disorganized, there will be a rough voice, whereas, if glottic closure is incomplete, the voice may be breathy. Superficial mucosal lesions may be congenital (sulcus vergeture), secondary to inflammation (cysts, sulcus vocalis,

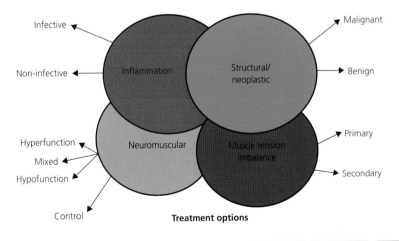

Figure 15.5 Aetiological categories of voice disorders and their interactions (With acknowledgement to Professor J. Koufman).

Table 15.2 Important points in patient history

- Voice problem, e.g. abnormal quality, pitch, loudness, loss of voice function
- Onset and duration
- Constant/intermittent
- Relieving and exacerbating factors
- Voice requirement in terms of fine precision and control, voice projection and continuous periods of use
- Social history, hobbies and lifestyle factors
- Smoking and alcohol consumption
- Dietary habits
- Caffeine and fluid intake

- Past and current medical history including conditions affecting the respiratory, gastro-oesophageal, neurological, musculoskeletal and endocrine systems
- Psychological and psychiatric conditions
- Effects of drugs*:
  - Reduced laryngeal secretions and mucosal drying, e.g. anti-cholinergics, diuretics
  - Irritant, e.g. bronchial inhalers
  - Androgenic , e.g. danazol
  - Predisposition to infection, e.g. candidosis from steroid inhalers
  - Predisposition to gastro-oesophageal reflux
  - Central nervous system, e.g. Parkinsonism secondary to anti-psychotics

*Frequently prescribed medications and effects on voice and speech can be found at www.ncvs.org/ncvs/info/vocol/rx.html

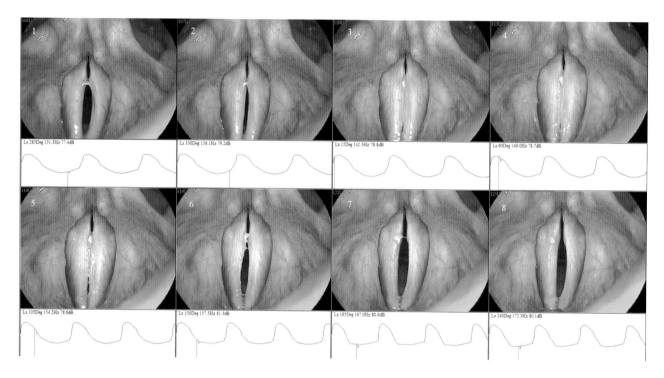

Figure 15.6 A series of images obtained using laryngostroboscopy taken at eight phases of the vibratory cycle and demonstrating the opening and closing of the glottis during phonation due to the mucosal wave motion.

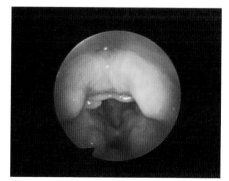

Figure 15.7 Marked laryngeal inflammation secondary to laryngopharyngeal reflux.

mucosal bridges, granulomas), due to surgical trauma (intubation, granulomas, scarring), or due to physical damage by voice abuse with inflammation (nodules, ectasia, polyps, pseudocysts, Reinke's oedema) (Fig. 15.9). Androgens can cause the female larynx to enlarge, and hypothyroidism can cause vocal fold thickening. The vocal fold and false cords may be distorted by neoplasms, deformities of the laryngeal skeleton or external trauma (Table 15.4).

The diagnosis usually follows videolaryngostroboscopy or microlaryngoscopy. In some cases, adequate improvement in vocal function is achieved with vocal hygiene, voice therapy and treatment of inflammation. Surgical resection is often required and microlaryngoscopy and biopsy should always be performed where malignancy is suspected.

Table 15.3 Treatment options for patients with voice problems

- Reassurance/education
- Vocal hygiene, lifestyle and dietary advice:
  - Stop smoking
  - Cut out excessive alcohol
  - Limit caffeine intake
  - Drink 1.5–2 litres of water/day
  - Reduce intake of fatty foods
  - Avoid eating within 3 hours of going to bed
  - Avoid irritants, e.g. dust, chemicals
  - Ensure atmosphere moist
  - Use steam inhalations
  - Avoid throat clearing
  - Avoid damaging voice through overuse by screaming/yelling or talking above background noise for prolonged periods
- Voice therapy:
  - Patient education
  - Relaxation techniques to reduce muscle tension
  - Improve efficiency of vocal function
  - Change vocal behaviour
  - Counselling
  - Laryngeal manual therapy
  - Advice on coping strategies
  - Advice on amplification aids
- Specialist therapy:
  - Singing lessons
  - Voice craft
- Medical treatment:
  - Antibiotics rarely effective
  - Antifungal medication if candidiasis suspected
  - Antireflux medication – proton pump inhibitor 1 hour before breakfast and evening meal for at least 2 months; alginates after meals and at night
  - Botulinum toxin injection for spasmodic dysphonia
- Surgery:
  - Phonosurgery/microlaryngoscopy (diagnostic; biopsy; glottoplasty)
  - Medialization surgery (laryngeal framework surgery; thyroplasty; injection techniques)
  - Transoral laser resection

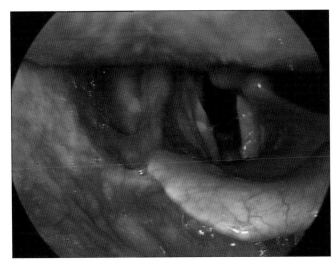

Figure 15.8 Left vocal cord palsy.

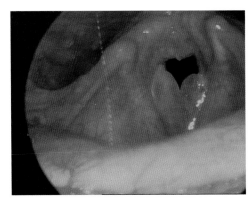

Figure 15.9 Example of structural abnormality: gross Reinke's oedema.

Inflammatory conditions

Inflammation of the larynx can be infective or non-infective (Table 15.5). In acute infection, laryngitis may be part of an upper respiratory tract infection, or secondary to rhinosinusitis or lower respiratory tract infection. Fungal infection by *Candida albicans* follows the incorrect use of steroid inhalers, or immunosuppression. Other causes of hoarseness in asthmatics are the drying irritant effects of some inhalers, muscle tension imbalance and laryngopharyngeal reflux.

Laryngitis may be non-infective – laryngopharyngeal reflux is one of the common causes. This is likely if hoarseness is worse in the morning and associated with other symptoms, such as chronic cough, phlegm in the throat, throat clearing, globus sensation and difficulty swallowing liquids and tablets. The diagnosis of laryngopharangeal reflux is usually made based on the history, laryngeal findings, exclusion of other causes and response to a therapeutic trial of antireflux medication (Table 15.3). The absence of heartburn does not exclude laryngopharangeal reflux as a cause.

Physical trauma, due to increased friction between poorly lubricated vocal folds, prolonged shouting, inadequate fluid intake, dehydrating agents or exposure to external irritants, can also cause laryngitis.

The changes seen in laryngitis range from a few prominent vessels on the vocal folds to gross oedema, erythema, ulceration or leucoplakia of the whole laryngopharyngeal mucosa. Stroboscopy is used to determine stiffness of the mucosa of the vocal fold on vibration.

Table 15.4 Structural or neoplastic conditions

- Benign:
  - Mucosal deposits/thickenings
  - Nodules
  - Polypoid nodules
  - Reinke's oedema
  - Pseudocyst
- Deficits/tethering:
  - Cysts
  - Epidermoid
  - Mucus retention
  - Sulcus vocalis
  - Sulcus vergeture
  - Mucosal bridge
  - Scarring
- Microvascular lesions:
  - Ectasia
  - Haemorrhagic polyp

- Malignant/premalignant:
  - Epithelial (hyperkeratosis, dysplasia, SCC, neoplasms)
  - Minor salivary gland
- Endocrinological:
  - Hypothyroidism
  - Androgenic
- Inflammatory mass:
  - Papillomatosis
  - Granuloma (arytenoids or pyogenic)
  - Rheumatoid deposits
  - Amyloid
- Laryngeal framework trauma
- Laryngoceles
- Mixed/reactive

SCC, squamous cell carcinoma.

Table 15.5 Inflammatory causes

Infective	Non-infective

Primary:
• Laryngeal – viral, bacterial (including tuberculosis) or fungal, e.g. *Candida albicans*
Secondary:
• Pulmonary infections
• Rhinosinusitis
	• Laryngopharyngeal reflux
	• Allergy
	• Trauma/irritation:
	  • Physical, e.g. phonotrauma
	  • Fumes/chemical
	  • Smoke
	  • Laryngeal dehydration
	• Drugs:
	  • Direct irritant, e.g. asthma inhalers
	  • Indirect, e.g. antimuscarinics
	• Autoimmune, e.g. Sjogren's syndrome
	• Non-specific

Absence of a mucosal wave suggests infiltration by carcinoma or tuberculosis.

Infective cases may settle after antibacterial or antifungal treatment. Non-infective laryngitis needs advice about voice use or rest, lifestyle and diet (Table 15.3). In non-responsive cases with impairment of mucosal waves, diagnostic microlaryngoscopy, including biopsy or incision and exploration of Reinke's space (cordotomy), is advisable.

Neuromuscular conditions

Neuromuscular conditions (Table 15.6) arise when the neural pathway or vocal muscles are impaired.

True hypofunctional conditions occur with global reduction in vocal muscular activity. The voice is weak, the pitch range reduced and the voice tires easily. Examples include Parkinson's disease, myasthenia gravis and bulbar palsy. Hyperfunction with speech tasks is seen in spasmodic dysphonia, which is a dystonia causing a staccato quality to the voice. Hyperfunction arises in pseudobulbar palsies, chorea and spastic dysphonia secondary to cerebrovascular accidents.

Table 15.6 Neuromuscular conditions

- Hypofunctional:
  - Parkinson's disease
  - Myasthenia gravis
  - Bulbar palsy
- Hyperfunctional:
  - Spasmodic dysphonia
  - Pseudobulbar/spastic dysphonia
  - Chorea

- Mixed or variable hypo/hyperfunctional:
  - Vocal cord palsy
  - Motor neurone disease
  - Multiple sclerosis
- Control/coordination:
  - Tremor
  - Myoclonus
  - Cerebellar lesions

Voice problems may be the first signs of more generalized neuromuscular disorder, such as Parkinson's disease, motor neurone disease, multiple sclerosis and myasthenia gravis. These should be considered in cases in which the vocal folds look normal, but the pattern does not fit a muscle tension dysphonia, fails to respond to voice therapy, or worsens progressively.

The voice in more general neurological conditions, such as Parkinson's and myasthenia gravis, may improve with systemic treatment for the underlying disease. Spasmodic and spastic dysphonia is often relieved for a few months by intralaryngeal injections of botulinum toxin. Unilateral palsies may respond to voice therapy, but they often need surgical medialization of the vocal cord. This is achieved by injecting a material, such as autologous fat or a polymethylsiloxane elastomer, into the vocal cord.

The commonest neuromuscular conditions are unilateral vocal cord palsies from recurrent laryngeal, superior laryngeal or vagus nerve damage. Viral neuropathy may account for 'idiopathic cases'. Patients with a palsy complain of weak voice, effortful phonation, throat discomfort or vocal fatigue as the vocal folds fail to meet, and there may be choking episodes as a consequence of glottic incompetence. Laryngeal examination reveals immobility of the vocal cord. Stroboscopy exposes asymmetry of phase and amplitude of the mucosal wave and apparent bowing on the affected side (Fig. 15.6).

Muscle tension imbalance conditions

This manifests as imbalance between specific synergists and antagonists or between one side of the larynx and the other, or as a global

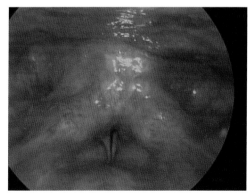

Figure 15.10 Example of muscle tension imbalance showing marked supraglottic constriction.

Table 15.7 Muscle tension imbalance

Primary	Secondary

• Vocal demands/strain:
  • Occupational
  • Inadequate vocal skills
• Psychogenic:
  • Anxiety/stress
  • Conversion dysphonia/
    aphonia
• Puberphonia/mutational
  voice disorder
	• Inflammation, including post-infection
	  problems
	• Structural/neoplastic, including end-stage
	  hyperfunction
	• Neuromuscular
	• Breathing disorders
	• Postural abnormalities
	• Congenital laryngeal anatomical
	  abnormalities
	• Presbylaryngis

increase in tension of the intrinsic and extrinsic laryngeal muscles (Fig. 15.10 and Table 15.7). Primary imbalance follows increased demands on the voice, or poor vocal technique. Poor posture and breathing patterns play a part.

Anxiety, stress and depression or conversion disorders are also causative factors. Tension imbalance also leads to structural abnormalities such as vocal fold nodules. The diagnosis of muscle tension imbalance is based on the history, listening to the voice, and response to vocal therapy exercises. Voice quality is variable and out of proportion to laryngeal findings.

Treatment (Table 15.3) includes reassurance, vocal hygiene advice and voice therapy.

Conclusions

Although a detailed history may point to a diagnosis, it is impossible to exclude malignancy or other physical abnormalities without a laryngeal examination. In primary care, the risk of malignancy needs to be carefully assessed and urgent referral made if it is a possibility. In other cases, with an obvious primary cause, simple lifestyle, vocal hygiene and dietary advice, or a therapeutic medical trial, is worth considering (Table 15.6). All other cases need referral for laryngeal examination. Laryngologists address key questions from the consultation (Box 15.4). Regional access to more specialized investigations and treatment should be available.

Box 15.4 **Questions to put forward at a consultation**

- What conditions (structural/neoplastic, inflammatory, neuromuscular and muscle tension imbalance) are present?
  - Can malignancy be excluded with certainty?
  - Are a microlaryngoscopy and biopsy required?
- What is the degree of certainty of diagnosis and how can that certainty be improved?
  - Are specialist tests or a trial of voice therapy or medical required?
- What are the primary conditions and what are secondary/compensatory? For example, muscle tension imbalance may be necessary to overcome poor glottic closure in a vocal cord paresis. A trial of voice therapy with muscle relaxation exercises may make the voice quality worse helping to confirm the diagnosis and indicating that a surgical medialization procedure would be the treatment of choice.
- What conditions are directly related to the patient's complaints? The most obvious condition may not be the primary cause of the patient's voice complaint. For example, inflammation or muscle tension imbalance may be more related to the patient's complaint rather than the thickened vocal folds in Reinke's oedema.

Further reading

Carding P. (2003) Voice pathology in the United Kingdom. *Br Med J*; **327**: 514–5.

Carding P, Hillman R. (2001) More Randomised Controlled Studies in Speech and Language Therapy. *Br Med J*; **323**: 645–6.

Carding PN, Horsley LA, Docherty GJ. (1998). The effectiveness of Voice Therapy for patients with non-organic dysphonia. *Clin Otolaryngol*; **23**(4): 310–18.

Jecker P, Orloff LA, Mann WJ. (2005). Extra-oesophageal Reflux and Upper Aerodigestive Tract Diseases. *ORL J Otorhinolaryngol Relat Spec*; **67**: 185–191.

Karkos PD, Thomas L, Temple RH, Issing WJ. (2005). Awareness of General Practitioners Towards Treatment of Laryngopharyngeal Reflux: A British Survey. *Otolaryngol Head Neck Surg*; **133**: 505–8.

National Center for Voice and Speech (1999) Frequently prescribed medications and effects on voice and speech. www.ncvs.org/ncvs/info/vocol/rx.html

Vaghela HM, Fergie N, Slade S, McGlashan JA. (2005) Speech therapist led voice clinic: Which patients may be suitable? *Logopedics Phoniatrics Vocology*; **30**(2): 85–9.

World Health Organization (1998) Towards a common language for functioning and disablement. Report ICIDH-2. WHO, Geneva.

CHAPTER 16

Trauma, Injuries and Foreign Bodies

Archana Vats, Antony Narula, Patrick J Bradley

OVERVIEW

- Haematomas of the pinna and the nasal septum should be drained as an emergency to prevent cartilage destruction.
- Traumatic perforations of the tympanic membrane, the majority heal spontaneously and should be "left alone", bigger perforation may be repaired surgically if referred urgently.
- Trauma or injury causing a facial nerve paralysis should be referred to a specialist for evaluation, as surgical repair when indicated is likely to restore function.
- Nasal fractures, causing a cosmetic deformity should be manipulated within 3 weeks, to restore alignment, otherwise allow the bones to heal and the deformity may require a cosmetic rhinoplasty.
- Major neck injuries require stabilisation of their cervical spine, in case of associated injury, maintenance of an airway and then referral to hospital for evaluation of the injuries.
- Sharp foreign bodies in the throat, tend to lodge in the tonsils, posterior tongue or hypopharynx and may require a general anaesthetic for removal.
- Beware not all fish bones are radio-opaque.
- Minature batteries wherever they are lodged or placed – ear, nose or throat MUST be removed immediately, otherwise corrosive injury will follow and may result in complications.

Ear

Injuries to the ear
Pinna

A blow to the ear can result in a 'cauliflower ear', due to tearing of blood vessels causing a subperichondrial haematoma. Haematomas should be aspirated or evacuated through an incision as soon as possible, and a compression dressing should be applied for 5–7 days. If not drained properly, a fibrosis develops: the fibrotic tissue organizes into a mass, with new cartilage forming a 'cauliflower'-shaped appearance.

Traumatic perforations

Traumatic perforations may result from blows to the ear from the flat of the hand or falling from water skis flat onto the water's surface. Severe atmospheric overpressure from explosion can tear the drum. Cleaning the ear canal can perforate the drum, as can inexpertly performed syringing.

Perforation may cause audible whistling, decreased hearing and a tendency towards infection during colds (upper respiratory tract infection, URTI) or if water enters the ear canal. Many perforations are asymptomatic and do not require a surgical repair. Most acute perforations heal spontaneously, without any treatment, within a few weeks.

Temporal bone fracture/traumatic face palsy

Fractures are classically divided into longitudinal, transverse and mixed types, but with the advent of CT scanning these divisions are theoretical. Longitudinal fractures comprise 70–80%, transverse 10–20% and mixed 10%. The incidence of facial paralysis is approximately 25% for longitudinal fractures and 50% for transverse fractures. Temporal bone fracture, resulting from closed head trauma, is the most common cause, and is associated with a facial paralysis, such as from motorcycle accidents. Injuries to the face may damage the peripheral part of the nerve. Injury during otologic or parotid surgery is an important cause of traumatic facial paralysis.

The onset and progression of facial paralysis are very important in deciding management. Nerve transection injuries present with immediate onset of paralysis, and have a poor functional outcome. Haematoma injuries may develop slowly and have a more favourable prognosis. Associated hearing loss or vertigo suggests the presence of a temporal bone fracture.

Initial evaluation may be delayed until more life-threatening injuries are treated. Particular attention should be given to any impairment of facial nerve function at presentation. Otoscopic examination of the external auditory canal (EAC) may reveal a step deformity of the bony canal or bleeding from a lacerated canal wall. Examination of the tympanic membrane and middle ear may show a haemotympanum (blood behind an intact ear drum) or perforation. Clear aural discharge suggests cerebrospinal fluid (CSF). Nystagmus occurs from vestibular system injury, and is another possible sign of temporal bone fracture. Tuning fork tests can easily be performed in an emergency department to corroborate the presence of conductive or sensorineural hearing loss. Conductive hearing loss is more commonly associated with longitudinal temporal bone fracture and sensorineural loss with a transverse fracture.

Most patients with intratemporal trauma, causing facial paralysis, recover some degree of function over time – usually months. With incomplete paralysis, the likelihood of full recovery of facial function is excellent. Patients with immediate onset of a complete facial paralysis probably have a poorer prognosis, but some recovery may

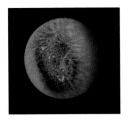

Figure 16.1 Foreign body in the ear canal.

still occur. Electrophysiology testing, when performed, suggests a favourable prognosis in patients with little degeneration within 14 days of the injury. Most patients without poor prognostic factors are likely to recover normal or near-normal facial nerve function.

A high-resolution CT scan of the temporal bone reveals multiple fracture lines in most cases, and may show bony fragment impingement on the facial canal.

Eye care with artificial tears and night patching should be implemented if upper eyelid function is impaired.

Surgical intervention is advocated, and can involve decompression of the facial nerve, possibly all the way from the internal acoustic canal to the stylomastoid foramen. In the case of nerve transection, if primary repair is not possible, a re-routing procedure or graft can be used.

Foreign bodies

Aural foreign bodies may present as incidental findings on otoscopy, or with otalgia, otorrhoea and hearing loss. They are most frequent in children under 10 years. Removal is rarely urgent. Insects in the external auditory canal can be drowned promptly, with the use of either alcohol or oil. Patients are best managed under the operating microscope in the ENT emergency clinic, with removal by suction, irrigation or microforceps (Fig. 16.1).

Rarely, if a large object is lodged deep in the ear canal, medial to the bony isthmus, or associated with otitis externa, the process may be so severe that the meatus is very narrow or closed. Here, a general anaesthetic may be required.

Nose

Nasal fractures

Long-term functional and cosmetic problems may follow if nasal fractures are not properly managed. Treatment of the long-term consequences is difficult. External nasal deformities and airway obstruction may follow inadequate management. The deformity depends on the direction of force applied. Forces from below may cause a complex pattern with fracture and dislocation of the septum.

The mechanism of injury should be recorded. The patient may note a change in nasal appearance. Anaesthesia, decongestion, lighting, suction and endoscopic equipment are necessary for internal examination. Laceration, ecchymosis, haematomas, mucosal tears and epistaxis internally strongly suggest fracture. Septal haematomas should be drained as soon as possible and the nose packed to prevent cartilage necrosis and the likely resultant saddle nose deformity.

The initial evaluation is often limited because of swelling. Once other injuries have been excluded and, if the patient is stable, then physical examination should be repeated after 5–7 days. The avail-

ability of previous photographs of the patient is helpful to identify pre-existing deformities.

Reduction of a nasal fracture is indicated in any patient with significant cosmetic deformity or functional compromise. This can wait no longer than 10 days, during which oedema resolves and positioning of the fractured bones correctly with more stability is easier. If reduction is not possible within the first 10 days, the fractured segments begin to form a fibrous union, which makes manipulation very difficult. The fractured segments are no longer mobile after 3 weeks. Full healing should be awaited (several months) before performing corrective rhinoplasty.

Imaging studies are rarely needed to evaluate traumatized nasal structures. The diagnosis is made on physical examination. CT scan is unnecessary, unless more serious injuries of the facial skeleton are suggested.

Manipulation under anaesthesia is performed by applying controlled external force to the deformed bones. These manoeuvres often adequately reduce associated displaced septal fracture. If this does not provide a satisfactory reduction, an instrument such as Asch forceps may be introduced with one blade in each nostril, or with one in the nostril and one outside, to reduce the fractured segment. A definitive rhinoplasty may be required.

Foreign bodies

Nasal foreign bodies may present acutely or even after years. They are found most commonly amongst toddlers and usually lodge between the septum and inferior turbinate – often visible on anterior rhinoscopy.

Organic material

Organic materials such as tissue paper, sponge or nuts, provoke an intense inflammatory reaction from the nasal mucosa. They are removed by grasping the object firmly with crocodile forceps or by passing a blunt hook distal to the foreign body and slowly withdrawing it forward, allowing for its removal.

Inorganic material

Inorganic material, for example a bead or button, requires careful removal by inserting a wax hook behind the object and sweeping forwards along the floor of the nose. A small suction catheter may withdraw objects such as polystyrene beads. Care should be taken not to let the child swallow the object as it is delivered from the nasal cavity. One attempt at removal is usually possible before the child becomes uncooperative and the use of a general anaesthetic is required.

Subacute presentation

Subacute presentation is the presence of a unilateral, foul-smelling nasal discharge, with excoriation of the vestibular skin. This should be considered as a foreign body until proven otherwise and may require examination of both nasal cavities under general anaesthetic.

A **battery** inserted into the nasal cavity requires urgent examination under general anaesthesia with a good light source, as its leakage occurs within hours resulting in corrosive burns and possible destruction of the nasal septum and inferior turbinate. Corroded mucosa should be irrigated with normal saline and inflamed mucosa treated with Naseptin cream.

Late presentation

In adults, retained foreign bodies present with unilateral nasal congestion and discharge, sometimes with sinusitis. A radio-opaque foreign object, when present, is demonstrable on CT scan. Calcium and magnesium carbonates and phosphates deposit around the foreign body forming a rhinolith, which must be extracted under general anaesthesia.

Neck

Penetrating neck trauma

Penetrating neck trauma is a rising cause of injury and death. Mandatory exploration used to be the recommended treatment and the mainstay of management in most major trauma centres. The concept of elective management was introduced in the 1980s because, although operative mortality rates were declining, the number of explorations with negative findings was rising. The most common causes are bullets and stab injuries. Stabbing usually results in less severe injury than missile wounds. Accidental injuries, with penetration of the platysma by a foreign object of metal, glass or wood, do not result in extensive collateral tissue damage, but foreign bodies may remain in the neck.

Penetrating neck wounds can cause injury to any of the major organ systems of the neck – the great vessels, larynx and trachea, oesophagus and spinal column – with 20–30% resulting in laryngeal, tracheal or oesophageal injuries.

A rapid assessment of the airway, breathing and circulation must come first. Expanding haematoma, subcutaneous emphysema, hoarseness, stridor, respiratory distress, haemoptysis and haemodynamic instability all suggest injury to the airway and/or vasculature. The approach to airway management must be individualized. A seemingly stable airway can be lost rapidly. With injury to the laryngotracheal complex, intubation can be attempted, but great care must be taken to recognize tracheal disruption. A marginal airway may be lost if intubation is not performed expertly. Significant trauma to the larynx or cricoid requires tracheostomy. Controlled tracheostomy with local anaesthesia is always preferred to an emergency procedure after unsuccessful intubation attempts.

Physical examination of the patient should focus initially on evaluation of the airway and respiratory status. The patient should be asked about changes in voice. The neck and upper chest should be palpated for subcutaneous emphysema, and the larynx and trachea for tenderness and crepitus. Flexible laryngoscopy, CT imaging and/or direct laryngoscopy and bronchoscopy may be necessary for full evaluation. Injuries to the great vessels of the neck may be obvious on physical examination, presenting as an exsanguinating wound or an expanding haematoma. Suspected vascular injuries can be evaluated further with angiography and exploration. Embolization techniques may be used to control bleeding, especially in inaccessible areas such as the base of the skull. Injuries to the oesophagus and pharynx are easily missed during the management of other immediately life-threatening injuries. Bleeding from the mouth, drooling and subcutaneous emphysema all suggest upper digestive tract injury.

Most vascular injuries in the neck will present within the first 48 hours, with delayed bleeding, or later with neurological deficit or haematoma formation. Patients with penetrating neck injuries need selective exploration.

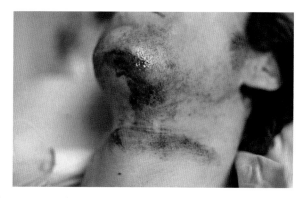

Figure 16.2 Crush injury to the neck region: fractured larynx.

Blunt neck injuries

These are common, and most are not associated with morbidity apart from bruising. However, blunt trauma to the larynx may produce multiple fractures of the thyroid cartilage (Fig. 16.2). Blunt injuries to the larynx are classified in order of severity, from minor bruising of the surrounding soft tissues, to minimal laryngeal fractures with no displacement but with internal mucosal tears, to gross laryngeal fractures with deformity, with or without pharyngeal or airway disruption. If laryngeal injury has been sustained or is suspected, and patients are asymptomatic, there may be little to find initially but, with time and local internal swelling, life-threatening airway obstruction may develop. Victims must be referred as emergency cases and evaluated by a laryngological expert. Management may involve tracheostomy and internal stenting of the larynx to restore the airway.

Throat/oro-hypopharynx

Foreign bodies

Patients with pharyngeal foreign bodies are usually adults, presenting acutely with pain and drooling. There is a lateralizing pricking sensation and significant dysphagia. Pharyngeal foreign bodies are commonly small bones and are not always radio-opaque. Small fish bones may lodge in the tonsil or tongue base and larger fish or meat bones in the hypopharynx. Visualization requires a good light, laryngeal mirror or a flexible nasendoscope. Tonsillar foreign bodies may be removed with a headlight and Tilley's forceps. Tongue base, vallecula and piriform fossa foreign bodies may be removed under local anaesthetic after generous application of Xylocaine spray. Indirect laryngoscopy with the patient sitting up, pulling the tongue forward using a swab, allows inspection with a warmed laryngeal mirror, and extraction using a McGill's forceps. Alternatively, the patient may be placed supine with the head below the horizontal in the surgeon's lap. A laryngoscope blade is used to control the tongue and the bone is removed under direct vision with a McGill's forceps. The patient should then not eat or drink until anaesthesia has worn off, at which time he or she may be discharged. Foreign bodies such as fish bones may be seen and extracted using forceps inserted into the instrument port of an endoscope. A flexible nasendoscope may be passed along the floor of the nose into the pharynx. Some patients require general anaesthesia.

On occasions, a lateral soft tissue radiograph of the neck may show a foreign body, such as coins and fish bones, which will require gen-

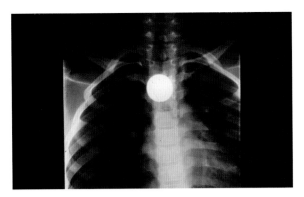

Figure 16.3 A coin visualized in the hypopharynx.

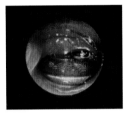

Figure 16.4 A coin lodged in the hypopharynx.

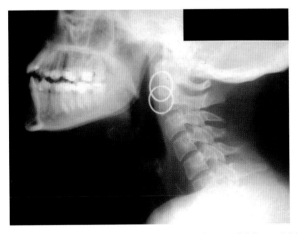

Figure 16.5 Acute presentation of foreign body in throat – fish bone visible in hypopharynx.

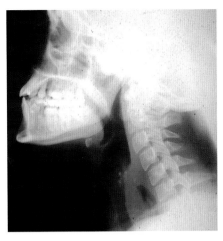

Figure 16.6 Same patient as in Fig. 16.5, 48 hours later, showing hypopharyngeal abscess with air and fluid level.

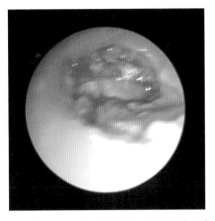

Figure 16.7 One battery lodged in the hypopharynx causing ulceration and erosion of the mucosa.

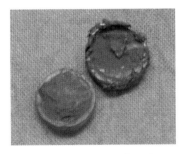

Figure 16.8 Same patient as in Fig. 16.7: two batteries removed by rigid endoscopy.

eral anaesthetic removal (Figs 16.3–16.6). One foreign body that requires immediate and urgent removal is the ingestion of a miniature battery, e.g hearing aid (Figs 16.7 and 16.8).

If no foreign body is visible and the patient is well and swallowing, with normal radiography, symptoms are likely to come from pharyngeal abrasion. The patient should be re-examined after 48 hours.

Tracheo-bronchus

Foreign body

Patients present in distress, with abnormal breath sounds, cough, wheeze, stridor or respiratory infection. Typical foreign bodies include coins, buttons, beads or organic material such as nuts and seeds, which may provoke an intense inflammatory reaction. There may be unilateral chest signs such as crepitation. A chest X-ray may show hyperinflation or hyperlucency.

Any child with respiratory difficulty after an episode of choking following play with small objects should undergo bronchoscopy by an experienced paediatric ENT surgeon and a senior anaesthetist. Objects usually lodge in the right main bronchus, as this is larger and more vertical than the left. Any foreign body must be grasped firmly and slowly withdrawn with the appropriate instrument (Fig. 16.9) The bronchi are gently cleaned of secretions afterwards.

There may be more than one foreign body, so all areas should be inspected. Adults and cooperative children can have bronchial foreign material retrieved under sedation with a flexible bronchoscope. This has an instrument port to allow insertion of flexible forceps,

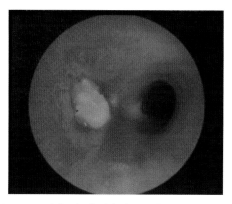

Figure 16.9 An organic foreign body lodged in the bronchus.

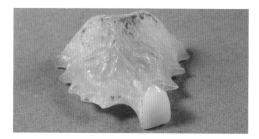

Figure 16.11 An upper denture with no radio-opaque markers.

which may be used to extract the material. Rarely, bronchial foreign bodies require thoracotomy by a cardiothoracic surgeon.

Oesophagus

Foreign bodies

Patients with oesophageal foreign bodies present with neck or chest pain, excessive salivation and dysphagia, often total. In children, the commonest object is a coin; in adults, bones or false teeth (Figs 16.10 and 16.11). A food bolus may impact in a normal oesophagus – above the cricopharyngeus, the arch of the aorta, the gastro-oesophageal sphincter – or wherever disease such as stricture or malignancy is present. Examination may be normal. Radio-opaque foreign bodies may be visible on lateral and anterposterior (AP) X-rays, or there may be an oesophageal air bubble, soft tissue swelling or surgical emphysema. Pharyngeal foreign bodies usually lodge at the narrowest point of the upper gastrointestinal tract – just above the cricopharyngeus muscle in the hypopharynx. Soft foreign bodies with no evidence of bone, such as meat boluses, may be managed medically with a muscle relaxant and anti-inflammatory drugs. Frequently the bolus may move on over 2 hours. The patient can be reassessed and, if then drinking normally, can be discharged. Those who remain symptomatic are managed either by gastroenterolo-

gists or ENT surgeons, with a flexible gastroscope advanced as far as the obstruction. All patients with food bolus impaction should undergo contrast swallow as an outpatient afterwards to ensure that there is no local disease to account for the incident.

Patients presenting with a history of a sharp foreign body, usually meat with bones, should not be given muscle relaxants or anti-inflammatories for fear of inducing a viscus perforation. Sharp foreign bodies require rigid oesophagoscopy under general anaesthesia by an ENT surgeon. Following rigid endoscopy, all patients should remain off oral ingestion for several hours and should be observed for symptoms and signs, such as pain, odynophagia, fever or tachycardia – features suggesting pharyngeal or oesophageal perforation, and possible mediastinitis (Fig. 16.12).

Further reading

Belleza WG, Kalman S. (2006) Otolaryngological emergencies in the outpatient setting. *Med Clin Nth Am*; **90**(2): 329–53.

Bernius M, Perlin D. (2006) Pediatric ear, nose and throat emergencies *Pediatr Clin North Am*; **53**(2): 195–214.

Lam HC, Woo JK, van Hasselt CA. (2001) Management of ingested foreign bodies: A retrospective review of 5240 patients. *J Laryngol Otol*; **115**: 954–7.

Mc Rae D, Premachandra DJ, Gatland DJ. (1989) Button batteries in the ear, nose and cervical oesophagus: a destructive foreign body. *J Otolaryngology*; **18**(6): 317–19.

Sosse RJ, Simons JP, Mandell DL. (2006) Evaluation and management of paediatric oropharyngeal trauma. *Arch Otolaryngol Head Neck* **132**: 446–51.

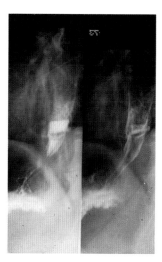

Figure 16.10 A contrast swallow demonstrating a foreign body in the lower oesophagus.

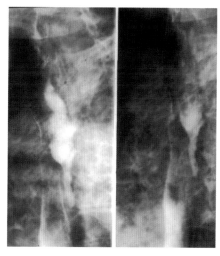

Figure 16.12 A contrast swallow of the oesophagus, showing surgical emphysema with a perforation (contrast outside the oesophagus) caused by the dentures in Fig.16.11.

CHAPTER 17

Epistaxis, Catarrh, Glossodynia, Halitosis and Somatization

Nick S Jones, Patrick J Bradley

OVERVIEW

- Epistaxis, the majority are a social nuisance and do not require treatment. Epistaxis in the elderly population may be profuse, dangerous and maybe associated with death, if not managed aggressively.
- Catarrh should be considered a symptom and not a disease as such, and may be defined as 'conscious awareness of mucus in the throat'.
- Glossodynia or "Burning Mouth Syndrome" requires that serious diseases need to be excluded, but the symptom may require psychiatric treatment.
- Somatising patients are commonly seen with ENT symptoms, as many as 25%, serious organic disease must be excluded with speed and minimal investigation.

Epistaxis

Nosebleeds range from a recurrent nuisance to major life-threatening events. The current worry about blood as a potential source of infection has increased the frequency of the scenario of parents repeatedly being called to fetch their child from school because of a nosebleed. Young children usually bleed from just inside the nose at the mucocutaneous junction, and this invariably stops spontaneously. Adults tend to bleed from Little's area (from veins) on the anterior third of the septum. Bleeding may arise from a maxillary spur near the floor of the nose, further back or higher up the septum. On occasion, there is a pathological process causing the problem; for example, patients on anticoagulants, those with bleeding diathesis or those with hereditary haemorrhagic telangiectasia. Dilated vessels can often be seen in Little's area (Fig. 17.1).

Sometimes there is a dry or crusted area. An event has damaged the cilia lining the nose and interfered with the self-cleansing clearance of mucus, leaving a raw base that may bleed. Nose-picking is common. A deviated septum or prominent maxillary spur may cause turbulence of air with drying, and the resulting crusts may bleed when dislodged. Some patients with allergic rhinitis suffer more nosebleeds in the hayfever season and topical nasal steroids often aggravate bleeding. It may be helpful for the patient to use the spray from the right hand for the left nostril and vice versa, so the spray does not hit the same area of septum each time.

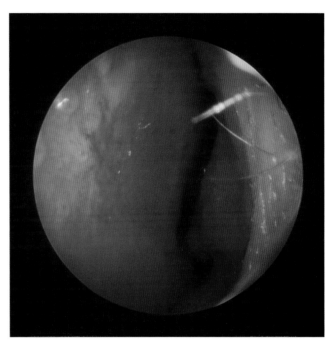

Figure 17.1 A vascular area on the left side of the septum in Little's area.

First aid measures include asking the patient to apply constant firm pressure over the lower (non-bony) part of the nose for 20 minutes, leaning forwards with the mouth open over a bowl to estimate blood loss. Blood dripping postnasally will be swallowed, and the next warning sign could be the vomiting of a large quantity.

It is important to estimate the loss. A cupful of blood on the floor is alarming but not dangerous in an adult, but daily this amount for a week may compromise an elderly person. Pulse and blood pressure measurements should be repeated as necessary. A fall in blood pressure is a late sign, particularly in young people, who can maintain their pressure by peripheral vasoconstriction despite a large blood loss. Measuring haemoglobin within the first 12 hours of a nosebleed does not give a reliable idea of blood loss, as there will have been no significant haemodilution.

If first aid measures do not work, the insertion of a nasal pack or dressing is considered. Some of these expand when wet, whilst others have haemostatic properties and dissolve. Non-dissolvable dressings should not be left in place for more than 36 hours because of the risk of toxic shock syndrome. About 15% of nosebleeds are not controlled by a pack. If bleeding is torrential, a postnasal pack or a posterior balloon catheter may be inserted, although this is unpleasant for the patient. With a postnasal pack in place, the patient must be admitted to hospital. A trained ENT surgeon should always examine the nose using suction and a light source to identify the site of the bleeding.

With a nasendoscope over 90% of nosebleeds can be identified and dealt with using suction bipolar diathermy. In many patients, it is possible to see a bleeding spot on Little's area, anaesthetize the area with a topical anaesthetic and vasoconstrictor, and then touch it with a silver nitrate stick or bipolar diathermy as an outpatient. Patients should be advised to keep the area moist by placing Vaseline just inside the nose from the end of their little finger, and 'milking' it around the affected area by gently squeezing their nostrils. This should be performed three or more times a day for 2 weeks to prevent any scab that forms drying and peeling off.

Rarely, in adult patients, if packing does not control the bleeding, the arterial supply from the maxillary artery or the anterior ethmoidal artery may need to be ligated, under general anaesthetic. External carotid artery ligation is very rarely performed nowadays. Embolization may be indicated for recalcitrant sufferers.

Catarrh and postnasal drip

'Catarrh' is a non-specific complaint with no precise definition. It may produce a sensation of mucus at the back of the throat or be associated with sniffing, snorting, clearing the throat repeatedly or hawking.

Anterior nasal discharge may be due either to overproduction of mucus, as in allergic rhinitis, or poorly functioning cilia in an upper respiratory tract infection. If posterior, there is a need to establish whether the patient has become over-aware of normal mucus, or whether there really is an overproduction.

The nasal mucosa may be overproductive in chronic rhinosinusitis, particularly in the presence of nasal polyps (Fig. 17.2). Habitual snorting or clearing the throat, in contrast, often accompanies hyperawareness of normal mucus. This activity maintains and exacerbates a sensation of mucus.

Often, a snorer with an oedematous uvula complains of 'something' around the soft palate, and describes it as 'catarrh' (Fig. 17.3). Some patients with globus pharyngeus may also complain of catarrh with a sensation of something (or mucus) at the level of the cricoid cartilage.

Many patients who mouth breathe during sleep wake with green-stained mucus that has collected in the naso- or oropharynx, as the mucus has dried there to become discoloured by oropharyngeal commensals or smoke particles. This may be suggested by the information that it becomes clearer throughout the day. If it is always discoloured, it is useful to ask them to blow into a handkerchief for inspection. Green mucus in a handkerchief suggests a chronic infective rhinosinusitis (Fig. 17.4). Patients with nasal polyposis often

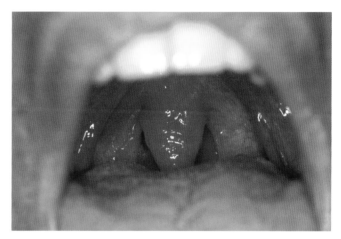

Figure 17.3 Some patients who incidentally snore and have an oedematous uvula complain of 'something' in their nasopharynx. They may habitually snort to try and clear this sensation.

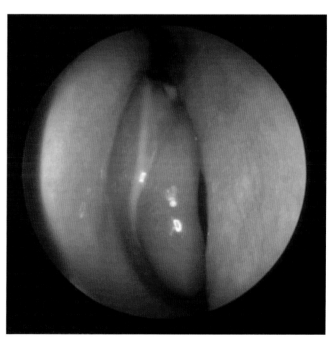

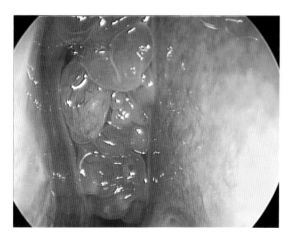

Figure 17.2 An endoscopic view of the right side of the nose showing nasal polyps.

Figure 17.4 An endoscopic view of the right side of the nose showing pus coming out of the paranasal sinuses.

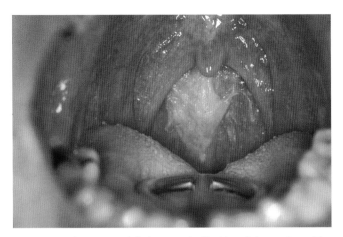

Figure 17.5 Clear postnasal discharge noticed incidentally in a patient with allergic rhinitis; there were no symptoms of postnasal discharge.

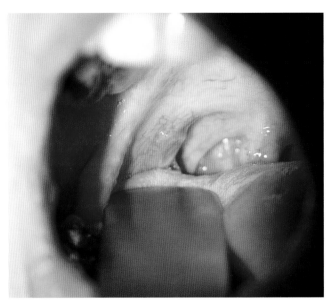

Figure 17.6 An aphthous ulcer on the right anterior pillar of the fauces that resolved within 10 days.

produce yellow-stained mucus, due to the presence of eosinophils. This discoloration does not mean that it is infected.

It is far more common for patients to have a hyperawareness of normal postnasal mucus and, through repeated clearing of their throat or snorting, to have 'sensitized' these areas to the half a cup of mucus that is normally produced from the paranasal sinuses each day, as well as the litre of saliva that is swallowed. In this context, it is worth considering that, of the large number of people with allergic rhinitis who have a definite increase in their mucus production, few complain of catarrh (Fig. 17.5).

The symptoms of postnasal drip syndrome (PNDS) are said to be those of 'something' dripping down from the nasopharynx, a need to clear the throat, a tickle in the throat, and posterior nasal discharge, therefore overlapping with the symptoms of catarrh. PNDS has been described as one of the 'pathogenic triad of the cause of chronic cough' together with asthma and gastro-oesophageal reflux. It has been suggested that the symptoms are due to mechanical stimulation in the upper airway and specifically due to secretions dripping into the hypopharynx. However, there is no clear definition and there is no physiological reason why secretions should 'drip' in this way – nasal mucus is normally tenacious and cannot drip. Most authorities in this field believe that nasal disease has a role in the production of chronic cough through a continuum or 'global' airway inflammation affecting the upper and lower airway. Non-specific pharyngeal symptoms on their own that have previously been attributed to PNDS do not usually suggest an indication of intranasal disease.

Burning mouth syndrome and glossodynia

Some patients complain of a persistently painful tongue that is typically not made worse by eating hot or spicy food. It often occurs in association with a dry mouth and there may be an alteration in the sense of taste.

It is important to exclude any causes of glossitis or stomatitis, although these are uncommon. If the papillae are lost and the tongue looks raw, check to see that there is no vitamin B_{12} deficiency or diabetes. If the oral mucosa has white plaques on it that can be scraped off, or under a patient's denture the mucosa looks raw and red, he or

she may have oral candida. This can occur when a patient has had one or several courses of antibiotics or in someone who is immunosuppressed. Variations in the number of papillae are not uncommon and can form a pattern called geographical tongue that is harmless. A raw area in the middle of the tongue with loss and/or discoloration of the papillae is median rhomboid glossitis, and this responds to antifungal treatment such as itraconazole. Other causes that must be excluded are a sensitivity to the dentures or a proprietary gargle, or a side effect of a drug. Lichen planus can take many forms but there is often an appearance of fine white striae in the posterior buccal mucosa, but it can cause erosions of the oral mucosa as well. Check for oral ulceration that may be due to the common minor aphthous ulcers (Fig. 17.6), or more indolent ulcers, such as major aphthous ulcers that not only have a larger diameter but persist for weeks, and those of Behçet's disease, mucous membrane pemphigus and malignancy.

If dryness is the primary symptom and this includes the eyes, then Sjögren's disease must be considered. The mucosa is often erythematous and sticky with atrophy of the filiform papillae.

Burning mouth syndrome is far more prevalent in postmenopausal women and in people who are depressed. Tricyclic antidepressants help to some extent, although these can compound the sensation of a dry mouth. More recently, gabapentin has been reported as helping some patients. Many patients are not helped by any medication and listening, support and information are all that can be offered. Somatization in the condition may be a factor.

Halitosis

Halitosis may be oral or extra-oral. Oral halitosis is the most common, being responsible for more than 90% of cases, with poor oral hygiene and periodontal disease as the primary culprits. Debris in tonsil pits can collect anaerobes in the extruded dead white cells, and this has an offensive smell. Oral malignancy can produce a foul anaerobic smell, so that the whole oral cavity including the posterior third of the tongue, the retromolar trigone and sublingual area should be inspected.

Extra-oral halitosis comes from the nose, the lower respiratory tract, blood-borne compounds exhaled, systemic diseases, metabolic disorders, medication and some foods. The paranasal sinuses are rarely a cause, except from anaerobic organisms collecting around a foreign body or rhinolith, or from dental infection that involves the maxillary sinus.

Somatization

Somatizing patients experience distressing symptoms that cannot be fully accounted for by organic disease, and they attribute their symptoms to a physical illness. Often the distress caused by the symptoms is out of proportion when compared to that of someone with organic disease, and there may be symptoms of depression and anxiety. In prevalence studies, approximately 25% of patients attending their general practitioner or ENT surgeon had somatization. Typical symptoms include a fullness in the head or ears, dizziness without vertigo, catarrh or a dry sore throat. There are often many recurrent symptoms that change in nature. It is common for these patients to seek many opinions. It is important to exclude any organic pathology that can present with these symptoms by performing a thorough examination and any relevant investigation. If the patient is thought to have somatization, it is important to then minimize the number of investigations, withdraw unnecessary treatment, address any psychological problems, and, whilst fully acknowledging the patient's symptoms, to give unambiguous reassurance. If the patient's ability to function is impaired by his or her condition, it may be necessary to seek psychiatric help.

Further reading

Bensing JM, Verhaak PF. (2006) Somatisation: a joint responsibility of doctor and patient. *Lancet*; **367**: 452–4.

Buchanan J. (2006) US6 Burning mouth syndrome *Oral Dis*; **12** (Suppl 1): 4

Monkhouse, WS, Davey, DA, Bradley, PJ. (1986) What do you mean by catarrh? *British Journal of Clinical Practice*; **40**: 417–20.

Murthy P, Nilssen EL, Rao S, McClymont LG. (1999) A randomised trial of antiseptic nasal carrier cream and silver nitrate cautery in the treatment of recurrent nasal epistaxis. *Clin Otolaryngol*; **24**(3): 228–31.

O'Hara JT, Jones NS. (2005) The aetiology of chronic cough: a review of current theories for the otolaryngologist. *Journal of Laryngology and Otology*; **119**: 507–14.

Pokupec-Gruden JS, Cekic-Arambasin A, Gruden V. (2000) Psychogenic factors in the aetiology of stomatopyrosis. *Coll Antropol*; **24** Suppl 1: 119–26.

Umapathy N, Quadri A, Skinner DW. (2005) Persistent epistaxis: what is the best practice? *Rhinology*; **43**: 305–8.

Scully C, Felix DH. (2005) Oral Medicine: Oral malodour. *British Dental Journal*; **199**: 498–500.

Scully C, Porter S. (2005) Halitosis. *Clin Evid*; **14**: 1704–8.

CHAPTER 18

Neck Swellings

Shahed Quraishi, Patrick J Bradley

OVERVIEW

- Neck swellings are common findings that present in all age groups from many causes, ranging from congenital to acquired pathology, from cysts, inflammatory, infective to neoplastic disease, encompassing any neck structures.
- In the community, the inflammatory lymph node is most common, whereas in hospital thyroid swelling or goitre is most frequently seen.
- It behoves all clinicians to understand the embryology and anatomy to aid in making the correct diagnosis thus allowing for appropriate management.
- There are more than 100 lymph nodes in each neck, and the other organs or glands are singular!
- Knowledge of patients age, associated symptoms and anatomical location of the lump, is key to proceeding to treatment in General Practice, or is an indication for referral for further investigation, including surgery.
- Neck lumps in adults (over 40 years) should be considered malignant or at least have malignancy excluded by examination of the mucosal surfaces of the head and neck.

Surgical anatomy of the neck

Several normal structures are palpable on neck examination. In females, the cricoid cartilage is often the most palpable laryngeal structure; in men, it is the thyroid cartilage. The mastoid tip is palpable behind the ear. Between the mastoid tip and the angle of the mandible, the transverse process of the C1 vertebra is sometimes palpable. The carotid bulb can be felt near the anterior border of the sternocleidomastoid muscle, at the level of the hyoid bone, and may be mistaken for an abnormal mass, especially when the two bulbs are asymmetrical.

The position of an abnormal nodal mass may suggest the source of the primary lesion due to a predictive lymphatic flow pattern. Cervical lymphatics have been divided into five anatomical regions in the anterior and posterior triangles of the neck.

Diagnosis

History

The first consideration is the patient's age (Table 18.1). In general, neck masses in children and young adults are more commonly in-

Table 18.1 Age in relation to possible diagnoses

	Child (0–15 years)	Young adult (16–35 years)	Adult (35+ years)
Congenital	Cystic hygroma Thyroglossal duct cyst	Branchial cysts	Very uncommon
Inflammatory	Very common	Less common	Rare
Salivary disease	Inflammatory	Sialolithiasis	Neoplasms
Thyroid disease	Uncommon	Usually endocrine Papillary carcinoma	Most often endocrine Other thyroid malignancies
Neoplastic	Rare	Lymphoma Metastases	Lymphoma Squamous cell carcinoma Metastases

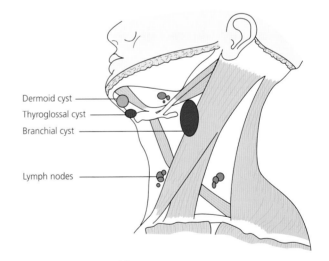

Figure 18.1 Common neck lumps.

flammatory than congenital, and rarely neoplastic. However, the first consideration in the late adult should be neoplastic. A 'rule of 80' provides a useful guide. In adults, 80% of non-thyroid neck masses are neoplastic, and 80% of these are malignant. A neck mass in a child, however, has a 90% probability of being benign.

The location of a mass is important (Fig. 18.1). Although congenital masses are more consistent in their locations, metastatic nodes follow a predictive pattern and help in identifying the primary malignancies.

The duration is one of the most important factors of history. Inflammatory disorders are usually acute in onset, and resolve within 2–6 weeks. Cervical lymphadenitis is often associated with recent upper respiratory tract infection. Congenital masses are often present from birth as small, asymptomatic masses, which enlarge rapidly after mild upper respiratory tract infection. Metastatic carcinoma tends to have a short history of progressive enlargement. Transient post-prandial swelling in the submandibular or parotid area suggests salivary gland duct stenosis that may lead to obstruction. Bilateral diffuse tender parotid enlargement is most commonly mumps in children and sialosis in adults.

Examination

Full head and neck examination (Table 18.2), including mucosal surfaces, is helpful, especially when suspecting malignancies. The oral and pharyngeal surfaces should be digitally palpated in addition to the neck mass. The location, mobility and consistency of a neck mass can often place it within a general aetiological group – congenital, nodal/inflammatory, vascular, salivary or neoplastic.

Congenital masses may be tender when infected, but are generally soft, smooth and mobile. A tender, mobile mass or a high suspicion of inflammatory adenopathy with an otherwise negative examination may warrant a clinical trial of antibiotics and observation for up to 2 weeks, with close follow-up. Chronic inflammatory masses and lymphomas are often non-tender and rubbery and may be either mobile or feel like matted adenopathy. In older age groups, the submandibular and parotid glands become ptotic and mimic neck lumps, and can cause concern to patients.

Diagnostic studies

- Full blood count and erythrocyte sedimentation rate (ESR).
- Viral serology: Epstein–Barr virus, cytomegalovirus and toxoplasmosis.
- Throat swab: occasionally helpful, but must be sent immediately in the proper medium.
- Thyroid function tests and ultrasound in all cases of thyroid enlargement.
- Chest X-ray in smokers with persistent neck lump.
- Fine needle aspiration biopsy (FNAB) is helpful for the diagnosis of neck masses and any neck lump that is not an obvious abscess and persists following antibiotic therapy. A negative result may require a repeat FNAB, ultrasound-guided FNAB or even an open biopsy.
- Ultrasonography is useful in differentiating solid from cystic masses.

- Radionuclide scanning: for suspected parathyroid and thyroid gland masses.
- Computed tomography (CT) scanning can distinguish cystic from solid lesions, define the origin and full extent of deep, ill-defined masses and, when used with contrast, can delineate vascularity or blood flow.
- Magnetic resonance imaging (MRI) is useful for parapharyngeal and skull base masses and for assessment for unknown primary carcinomas. With contrast it is good for vascular delineation, and MRI angiography may substitute for arteriography in the pulsatile mass or mass with a bruit or thrill.

Differential diagnosis according to position
Midline lumps
- Dermoid cysts;
- thyroglossal cyst (moves on protruding tongue);
- thyroid lump (moves on swallowing);
- lymphadenopathy.

Lateral neck lumps
- Submandibular triangle:
  - reactive lymphadenopathy (younger age group);
  - submandibular gland disease (sialadenitis, sialolithiasis, neoplasm).
- Anterior triangle:
  - reactive lymph adenopathy (younger age group);
  - neoplastic lymphadenopathy (firm, non-tender, older age group);
  - branchial cyst (second to third decades);
  - thyroid masses;
  - parotid gland disease (sialadenitis, cysts, sialolithiasis, neoplasm);

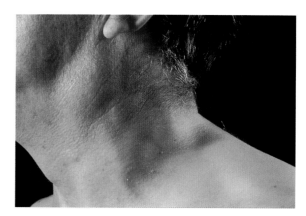

Figure 18.2 Laryngocoele (air-filled sac arising from laryngeal ventricle) in left neck on straining.

Table 18.2 Examination checklist

	Lymphadenitis	Branchial cyst	Goitre	Dermoid cyst	Thyroglossal cyst
Painful?	Yes	Possible	Possible	Possible	Seldom
Associated symptoms?	Yes	No	Yes	No	No
Moves with swallowing?	No	No	Yes	No	Yes
Midline?	Uncommonly	No	No	Yes	Yes
Moves on protruding tongue?	No	No	No	No	Yes

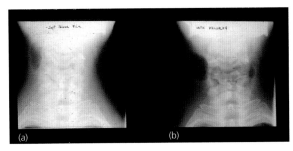

Figure 18.3 Radiograph: (a) at rest showing right-sided laryngocoele and (b) straining showing bilateral laryngocoeles (same patient).

- paraganglioma (carotid body tumour, glomus vagale);
- laryngocoele (enlarges with blowing) (Figs 18.2 and 18.3);
- cystic hygroma/lymphangioma;
- carotid bulb (in slender necks).
- Posterior triangle:
  - reactive lymphadenopathy (younger age group);
  - neoplastic lymphadenopathy (firm, non-tender, older age group);
  - lipoma;
  - cervical rib.

Characteristics of non-malignant neck lumps

Haemangiomas and lymphangiomas

These are congenital lesions usually present within the first year of life. Lymphangiomas usually remain unchanged into adulthood (Fig. 18.4), but haemangiomas (Fig. 18.5) most often resolve spontaneously within the first decade. A lymphangioma mass is soft, doughy and ill-defined, and may present with pressure effects. Haemangiomas often appear bluish and are compressible. CT or MRI may help define the extent of the neoplasm (Fig. 18.6), especially intrathoracic. Treatment of lymphangiomas includes injection with picibanil or excision for easily accessible lesions or those affecting vital functions. For haemangiomas, surgical treatment is reserved for lesions with rapid growth involving vital structures, which fail medical therapy.

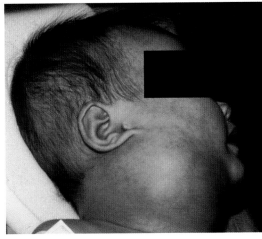

Figure 18.4 Lymphangioma in the parotid region.

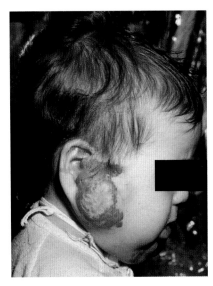

Figure 18.5 Haemangioma.

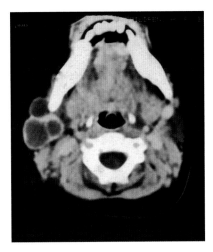

Figure 18.6 CT of lymphangioma.

Sebaceous cysts

These are common masses occurring most often in older people but can occur at any age. They are slow growing, but sometimes fluctuant and painful when infected. Diagnosis is made clinically; the skin overlying the mass is adherent and a punctum is often identified. Excisional biopsy confirms the diagnosis.

Branchial cleft cysts

A branchial cyst (Fig. 18.7), most commonly of second arch origin, usually presents as a smooth, fluctuant mass underlying the anterior border of the sternomastoid muscle. It often seems to appear rapidly after an upper respiratory tract infection as a tender mass. Occasionally, purulent material may be expressed if a sinus tract is present. These masses most commonly occur in the second or third decades. Primary treatment is with control of infection by antibiotics, followed by surgical excision.

Thyroglossal duct cyst

This is a common congenital midline neck mass (Fig. 18.8). It may

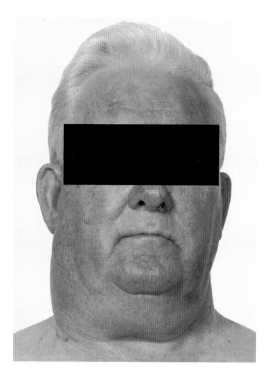

Figure 18.7 Branchial cyst.

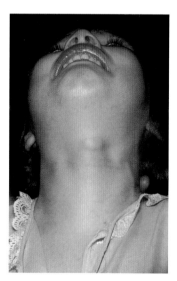

Figure 18.8 Thyroglossal duct cyst at level of hyoid bone.

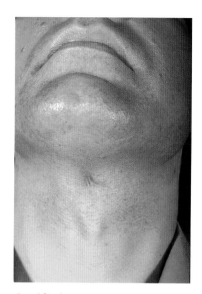

Figure 18.9 Thyroglossal fistula.

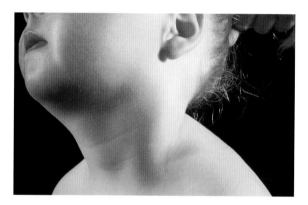

(a)

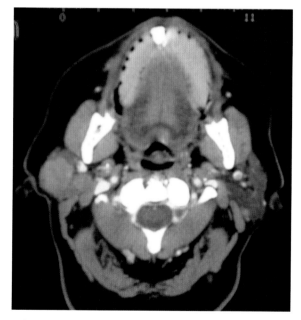

(b)

Figure 18.10 Cervical adenopathy: (a) mass in upper neck and (b) CT scan of neck mass.

sometimes be off centre at the lateral edge of the thyroid cartilage, and elevates on protrusion of the tongue. This distinguishes it from other midline masses, such as dermoid cysts or lymph nodes. Treatment is with initial control of infection with antibiotics, followed by surgical excision including the mid-portion of the body of the hyoid bone (Sistrunk's procedure). Occasionally, these lesions may become infected and resolve, or persist following surgery as a thyroglossal fistula (Fig. 18.9).

Lymphadenitis

Acute lymphadenitis is a common occurrence during the first decade. The presentation with a tender swelling, odynophagia, trismus and occasional torticollis with systemic signs of infection is a challenge

needing swift treatment with antibiotic therapy (Fig. 18.10). Less acute inflammatory nodes generally regress in size over 2–6 weeks.

If the lesion does not respond to conventional antibiotics, a biopsy is indicated after complete head and neck work-up to rule out malignancy or granulomatous disease. The rule of thumb is if a neck mass in an infant or child is bigger than a 'golf ball' after 3–4 weeks of observation or a course of antibiotics, then a serious underlying disease needs to be excluded – lymphoma or sarcoma.

Granulomatous lymphadenitis

These nodes usually develop gradually with slight symptoms over weeks and months. The glands tend to be firm, with some degree of fixation and infection of the overlying skin; radiology of the neck will demonstrate dystrophic calcification if tuberculosis is present (Fig. 18.11). They may suppurate and drain, only to re-form. Atypical mycobacteria and cat-scratch disease are more common and more prevalent in children, and may present in the parotid region (Fig. 18.12), or in the neck. Atypical mycobacterial infection usually involves anterior triangle lymph nodes often with brawny skin, induration and pain, whereas cat-scratch commonly involves the preauricular or submandibular nodes. Typical tubercular lymphadenitis often responds to anti-tuberculosis medications. Cat-scratch often undergoes spontaneous resolution with or without antibiotic treatment. Atypical mycobacterial infection may respond to combination antimicrobials or to complete surgical excision.

Lipoma

Lipomas are the most common benign soft tissue neoplasm in the neck. They are poorly defined, soft masses usually presenting after the fourth decade. They are usually asymptomatic, soft to feel and deep to the skin. FNAC or MRI Scan can confirm the diagnosis. Surgery is indicated when the lump is increasing in size, cosmesis, or when there is doubt about the accuracy of diagnosis.

Salivary tumours

Any enlarging mass at a radius of 5 cm from the angle of the mandible should raise suspicion for a primary parotid gland neoplasm, 80% of which are benign. Benign tumours are usually slow growing and asymptomatic; however, rapid growth, facial nerve palsy, cervical adenopathy, skin fixation or pain suggests malignant disease. Fine needle aspiration cytology (FNAC) helps to plan management and counselling in patients in whom malignancy is suggested. Ultrasound or MRI correlation helps to differentiate parotid cysts, intra-parotid lymph nodes, lipomas and localized sialadenitis from suspected neoplastic lesions (Fig. 18.13). For a definitive diagnosis, open excisional biopsy, either parotidectomy or submandibular gland excision, may be necessary.

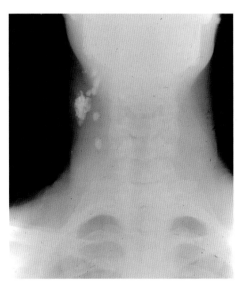

Figure 18.11 Radiograph of neck showing dystrophic calcification – tuberculosis.

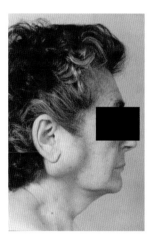

(a)

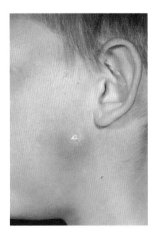

Figure 18.12 Atypical mycobacteria.

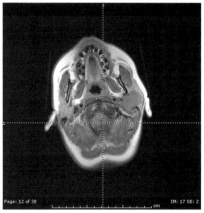

(b)

Figure 18.13 (a) Large parotid pleomorphic adenoma and (b) axial MRI scan.

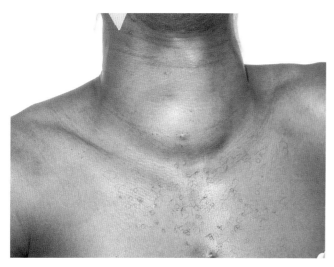

Figure 18.14 Thyroid mass.

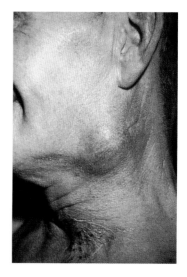

(a)

Thyroid masses

Thyroid neoplasms are a common cause of anterior compartment neck masses in all age groups, with a female predominance, and are mostly benign (Fig. 18.14). Fine needle aspiration of thyroid masses has become the standard of care and ultrasound may show whether the mass is cystic. Unsatisfactory aspirates should be repeated, and negative aspirates should be followed up with a repeat FNAC and examination in 3 months' time.

Paraganglioma (carotid body tumour, glomus vagale)

These are rare tumours usually found in adults. They are slow-growing painless lumps that have an average presentation at the fifth decade (Fig. 18.15). Sometimes they present as a parapharyngeal mass pushing the tonsil medially and anteriorly, or as a firm mass in the anterior triangle of the neck. Biopsy is contraindicated and MRI angiography is the investigation of choice. Surgical removal is based on patient factors and presenting symptoms.

Indications for specialist referrals

In the primary care setting, neck lumps are mostly caused by inflammatory conditions that are self-limiting, resolving within 2–6 weeks. A course of suitable antibiotics with a 2-week follow-up assessment is an appropriate first line of management. Failure to resolve requires hospital referral, especially if any presenting signs or symptoms suggest possible underlying malignancy. In a high-risk patient for malignancy with a neck lump, immediate referral is recommended; these are usually adults who have a history of smoking or chewing tobacco and indulging in excessive drinking of alcohol. Patients with lumps associated with weight loss or dysphonia (hoarseness),

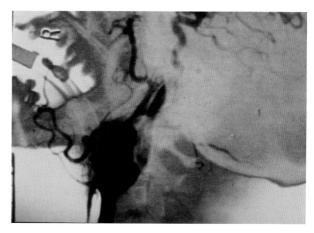

(b)

Figure 18.15 Carotid body tumour (paraganglioma): (a) clinical mass and (b) angiogram.

dysphagia (difficulty in swallowing), or dyspnoea (difficulty in breathing) for three or more weeks should be referred urgently for a head and neck assessment.

Further reading

Amedee RG, Dhurandhar NR. (2001) Fine needle aspiration biopsy. *Laryngoscope*; **111**(9): 1551–7.

Homer JJ, Silva P. (2003) Management of neck lumps. *Practioner*; **247**(1650): 726–34.

Mahoney EJ, Spiegel JH. (2005) Evaluation and management of malignant cervical lymphadenopathy with an unknown primary tumour. *Otolaryngologic Clinics of North America*; **38**(1): 87–97, viii–ix.

Umapathy N, De R, Donaldson I. (2003) Cervical lymphadenopathy in children. *Hospital Medicine*; **264**(2): 104–7.

CHAPTER 19

Head and Neck Cancer

Patrick J Bradley

OVERVIEW

- Head and neck cancer are increasing in incidence as the population ages.
- Squamous cell carcinoma of the mucus membrane is the most common cancer identified in the head and neck.
- Head and neck squamous cell carcinoma is no longer exclusively associated with excessive use of alcohol and smoking, younger patients non-drinking non-smoking are presenting more frequently in the last decade.
- The most common sites identified in the UK population, is the oral cavity and the larynx.
- Oral cavity cancer presents most common on the lateral border of the tongue, with ulceration and pain.
- Larynx cancer, most frequently presents with painless hoarseness because of involvement of the vocal cord (glottis).
- Patients diagnosed and treated for a head and neck cancer are at risk of developing a second primary head and neck cancer, the risk is estimated at 4% per year.

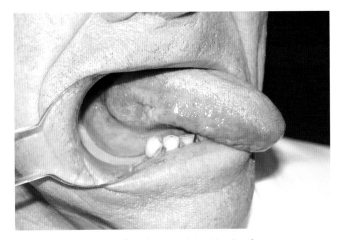

Figure 19.1 Squamous cell carcinoma on lateral border of tongue.

Definition

This subject is colloquially described as malignant tumours between 'the dura and pleura', or, more simply, all tumours/neoplasms of the mucous membrane and supporting tissues of the head and neck region, apart from the skin. Most (90%) are squamous cell carcinomas (Fig. 19.1). In the UK population, common sites are the oral cavity and the larynx (60–70%). Other sites include the nasal cavity, pharynx and middle ear, but also salivary and thyroid glands. Rarer tumours arise from soft tissues, bones and cartilages. Other cancers, such as lymphoma, may present in the head and neck region (Table 19.1 and Fig. 19.2) or as metastases from breast, lung, kidney and prostate.

Incidence

Globally, as well as within the European Union (EU), combining both sexes, cancer of the mouth and pharynx ranks sixth overall,

Table 19.1 Recorded numbers of new cases of head and neck cancer (all histological types) by country, sex and site, UK, 2000*.

Site	England Men/Women	Wales Men/Women	Scotland Men/Women	N. Ireland Men/Women	UK Men/Women
Oral cavity	1412/917	102/67	266/131	49/27	**1829/1142**
Larynx	1578/325	123/21	237/64	46/13	**1984/423**
Pharynx	1082/232	40/10	68/21	10/4	**1200/267**
Salivary gland	231/191	23/25	23/6	10/7	**287/239**
Thyroid gland	302/829	18/40	32/101	10/28	**362/998**
Total	**4605/2494**	**306/163**	**625/333**	**125/79**	

(*Toms JR (ed.) (2004) *CancerStats Monograph 2004*. Cancer Research UK, London.)

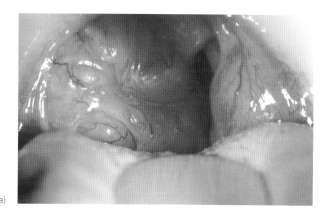

(a)

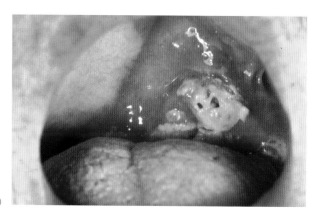

(b)

Figure 19.2 Malignant tonsil tumours: (a) non-Hodgkin's lymphoma and (b) squamous cell carcinoma.

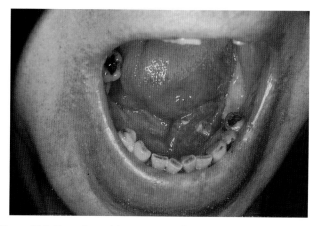

Figure 19.3 Floor of mouth in squamous cell carcinoma.

Symptoms and signs

Symptoms arise from local irritations, ulcerations and swellings. Ulceration in the oral cavity causes pain (Fig. 19.3). Swelling of the larynx produces hoarseness, breathing problems and local pain (Fig. 19.4). Soreness in the throat is the most common complaint with bleeding as the most uncommon presenting feature. National Institute for Clinical Excellence (NICE) Referral Guidance for suspected cancer lists the symptoms given in Box 19.1, which require specialist referral to a head and neck cancer clinic. These symptoms are non-specific and are frequent symptoms of many other disorders that affect the upper aero-digestive tract, and the reported cancer 'hit-rate' in such clinics is as low as 5–15%. Patients who present with such symptoms and do not respond rapidly to simple treatments, such as antibiotics, must be referred to exclude malignancy. Investigations of patients by general practitioners are not helpful in excluding head and neck cancer and often delay making the correct diagnoses.

There are several pre-malignant conditions. These include leucoplakia (white patch) (Fig. 19.5) and erythroplakia (red patch) (Fig. 19.6), and homogeneous, verrucous, nodular or speckled and mixed lesions. Potentially malignant conditions in the mouth include sideropenic dysphagia (mucosal atrophy associated with chronic iron-deficiency anaemia), erosive lichen planus, oral submucous fibrosis, discoid lupus erythematosus, tertiary syphilis and actinic keratosis. The term leucoplakia should be used for clinical description only and not as a substitute for histological diagnosis. Biopsy of such lesions is mandatory in predicting malignant potential. The risk of malignant transformation is around 3% per annum. Women who smoke are at higher risk. Patients do not have a decreased risk of malignant transformation even if the leucoplakia is treated. Dysplastic lesions, usually found at the glottic larynx, should be surgically treated if unifocal or easily removed. Radiotherapy may be considered if the lesion is multifocal or recurring frequently.

Uncommon head and neck cancers

Malignant salivary gland tumours are uncommon. The parotid gland is the most frequently affected, followed by the submandibu-

behind lung, stomach, breast, colon and cervix uteri, in that order. However, the mouth and pharynx is the third most common site for malignant disease in men in developing countries and the fourth in women. In the UK, there has been a 27% increase in oral cavity cancer cases from 3673 in 1995 to 4660 in 2003. Since 1989, the rate has steadily increased to reach 9.8 per 100 000 in 2003, an average increase of 2.2% each year since 1989. Altough female oral cancer rates have remained significantly lower than male rates, their incidence trends have been similar, with an average increase of 2.5% each year since 1989. However, there have been large increases in the incidence of oral cancer diagnosed in men in their forties and fifties, whose rates have doubled from 3.6 to 8.8 per 100 000 for men aged 40–49 and from 11.5 to 24.9 for men aged 50–59. The mortality rate from mouth cancer is just over 50% due to late detection. Despite treatment, there were 1679 deaths in 2004 – that is approximately one death every 5 hours. Larynx cancer is the fourteenth most common cancer in males, but is rare in females. There is a rising incidence in head and neck cancer and it is no longer exclusively associated with alcohol and smoking. People living in deprived areas are more likely to get head and neck cancer and are more likely to die than those in affluent areas. Thus the chances of survival are much improved if cancer is detected early and treated rapidly, but a majority present at a late stage. Advanced stage cancer is difficult to treat, with curative intent, and frequently leaves patients debilitated and disfigured.

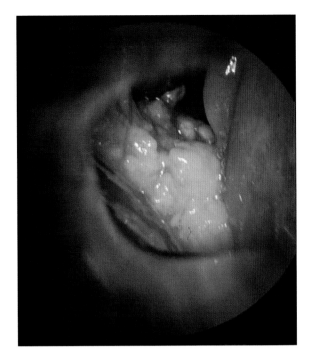
(a)

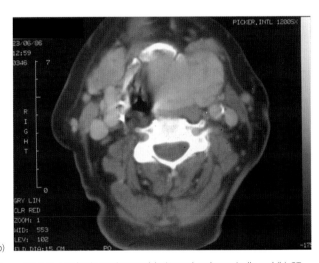
(b)

Figure 19.4 Supraglottic carcinoma: (a) pictured endoscopically and (b) CT scan to demonstrate extent of tumour size.

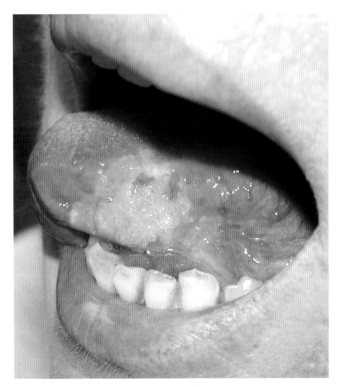

Figure 19.5 Leucoplakia on lateral border of tongue.

lar. In the majority of cases, the tumour presents as a slowly-growing painless mass in portions of the gland, as distinct from the whole gland being swollen or enlarged as in benign inflammatory disease. The association of a rapid increase in size, with pain, facial nerve paralysis and lymph node metastases, is uncommon now when compared with 20 years ago.

Patients presenting with swollen or enlarged thyroid glands are common in general practice, but the incidence of malignancy is low (Fig. 19.7). Patients who experience difficulty with breathing, with a swelling in the midline of the lower neck, must be referred urgently in case of a malignant thyroid compression syndrome. Other symptoms and associated factors (Box 19.2) must be sought, and such patients must be referred urgently to the local thyroid or head and neck clinic for investigation. Patients with a thyroid swelling without stridor or any other features should have thyroid function tests. Patients with hyper- or hypothyroidism and goitre are unlikely to have thyroid cancer and should be referred to an endocrinologist, or local thyroid expert. Patients with goitre and normal thyroid function tests should also be referred.

Risk factors

Head and neck cancer is rare in children under 16 years – nasopharyngeal and thyroid cancer being the most frequent. Other tumours

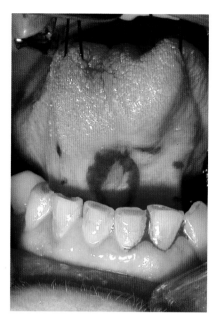

Figure 19.6 Erythroplakia on inferior portion of tongue.

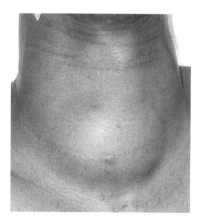

Figure 19.7 Enlarged thyroid swelling.

that can present in the paediatric age group include rhabdomyosarcoma, the most common soft tissue malignancy in children. This arises in any site but is found more often in the head and neck (40%) than any other region. Nasopharyngeal carcinoma is the most commonly misdiagnosed tumour of the head and neck because of local, regional and systemic symptoms either in combination or as isolated presentations.

Overall, mucosal head and neck squamous cell carcinomas, excluding skin cancers, represent about 6% of cancer incidence, and 5% of all cancer mortality. About 75% of these are of the oral cavity and pharynx and the remainder are laryngeal. In Europe, the incidence of oral and pharyngeal cancer and laryngeal cancer varies widely – it is highest in France, lowest in Greece. The lowest laryngeal cancer incidence is in the Netherlands. Men are at higher risk, usually aged between 40 and 70 years, reflecting social and recreational habits of different nations (Figs 19.8 and 19.9).

Cigarette smoking is the single most important risk factor in head and neck cancer. For the oral cavity in men, 90% of cancer risk can be

attributed to tobacco. Smoking attributable risk for laryngeal cancer in males and females is 80%. The relative risk of laryngeal cancer between smokers and non-smokers is 15.5 in men and 12.4 in women. Discontinuation of smoking reduces the risk of head and neck premalignant and malignant conditions. The risk of developing oral cancer by giving up for 1–9 years may be reduced by 30%, and by 50% by abstinence for over 9 years.

The association of alcohol with head and neck cancer is stronger for pharyngeal cancer than for any other head and neck site. Non-drinkers more often develop glottic than supraglottic cancer. The association between alcohol and cancer varies between oral cavity sites.

A synergistic effect of tobacco and alcohol on the development of head and neck cancers has been shown. The combined use of tobacco and alcohol increases the risk of laryngeal cancer by about 50% over the estimated risk of individual smoking or alcohol drinking (Table 19.2).

Other factors associated with head and neck cancers include chewing of the betel nut, poor dental hygiene, occupational exposure to materials such as hard wood, the development of adenocarcinoma of the paranasal sinuses and exposure to infective agents – human papillomavirus (HPV), human immunodeficiency virus (HIV), herpes simplex and Epstein–Barr virus.

Prognostic factors

Squamous cell carcinoma of the head and neck region is staged on the TNM system. T is tumour stage, N is cervical nodal stage and M is the presence or absence of distant metastases. The T stage defines the size of the primary tumour or the 'bulk involvement' of tumour to the local structures. The N stage, the clinical and pathological involvement of cervical lymph nodes, is:
• N0, the absence of cervical lymph involvement;
• N1, the involvement of a single node, less than 3 cm;
• N2a ipsilateral, single more than 3 cm;
• N2b ipsilateral, multiple, none more than 6 cm;
• N2c bilateral, or contralateral, none more than 6 cm;
• N3, the involvement of ipsilateral single nodal disease unilateral greater than 6 cm in greatest diameter.

The M status includes M0, no (known) distant disease, and M1, distant metastasis present – most frequently lung, liver or bone. It is possible to group these stages into 'early' and 'late' disease. Late

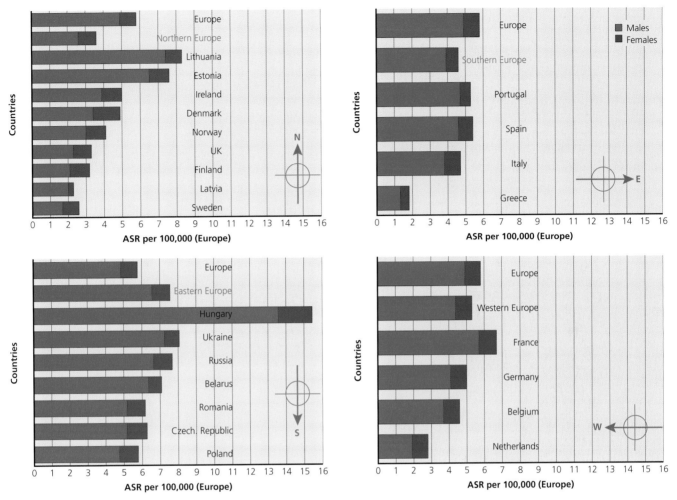

Figure 19.8 Age-related mortality rates in Europe, 1995, Cancer of the oral cavity. ASR, age-standardized rate.

disease involvement of local cervical lymphatics or local advanced disease is greater than T2 (Table 19.3).

Advanced disease has a worse prognosis than early, and is indicated by the presence of cervical nodal disease, the number and size of nodal disease involvement, and the level of nodal disease – the

Table 19.2 Relative risk of oral and pharyngeal cancer in men by cigarette smoking and alcohol consumption

	Drinks per week				
Cigarette smoking status	<1	1–4	5–14	15–29	30 or more
Non-smoker	1	1.3	1.6	1.4	5.8
Ex-smoker	0.7	2.2	1.4	3.2	6.4
1–19 daily for 20 or more years	1.7	1.5	2.7	5.4	7.9
20–39 daily for 20 or more years	1.9	2.4	4.4	7.2	23.8
40 or more daily for 20 or more years	7.4	0.7	4.4	20.2	37.7

Table 19.3 Staging of head and neck cancer (stage I and II, 'early'; stage III and IV, 'late')

Stage I	T1, N0, M0
Stage II	T2, N0, M0
Stage III	T1–3, N1, M0
	T3, N0, M0
Stage IV	T4, any N
	T1–3, N2–3
	Any T, any N, M1

lower the location in the neck, the worse the prognosis. Patients who present with a primary squamous cell carcinoma of the head and neck (called the index tumour), should they survive, have a risk of developing a second malignancy – the risk is estimated to be approximately 4% per year.

Most patients with head and neck squamous cell cancer are elderly, and many have coexistent, non-neoplastic (comorbid) diseases. Some comorbidities may be so severe that they can affect survival rates. They are referred to as prognostic comorbidity and include

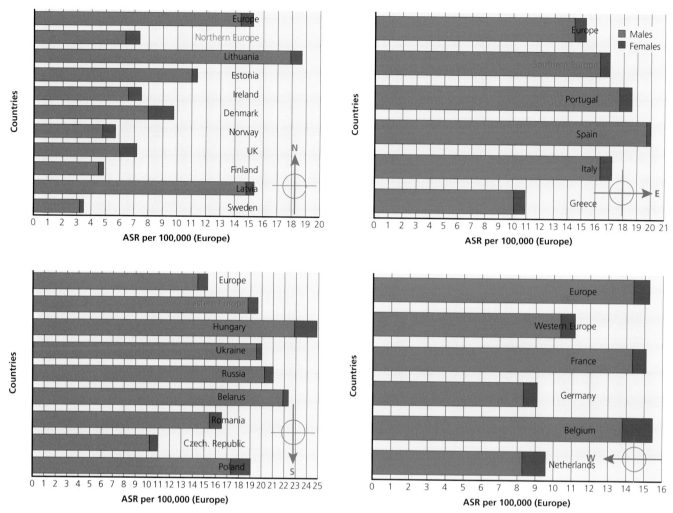

Figure 19.9 Age-related mortality rates in Europe, 1995, laryngeal cancer. ASR, age-standardized rate.

recent myocardial infarction, severe hypertension, severe hepatic disease, diabetes mellitus and severe weight loss. The Adult Comorbidity Evaluation-27 Index (ACE-27) is a validated instrument, and has been widely used in head and neck cancers.

Staging and evaluation

With all the information from examination, biopsy confirmation of a cancer and advanced radiological imaging, patients should be staged according to the TNM classification. In the UK, as in most countries, the process of patient management is presented and discussed in a forum of the Multidisciplinary Head and Neck Clinic Team (MDT).

Management of oral cavity cancer

In the UK, surgery is currently the treatment of choice for all oral cavity cancers, with postoperative radiotherapy when the pathological factors are unfavourable. Radiotherapy alone may be used for small tumours, or chemoradiotherapy for advanced inoperable tumours. The use of postoperative radiotherapy is frequently

required when the pathology reports perineural and/or perivascular involvement at the primary site, when there is the presence of extracapsular spread of cancer in the neck specimen, or when there is more than one lymph node involved. Free tissue transfer, most frequently the radial forearm flap, is used to replace surgically removed tissue, to preserve tongue mobility, and to enhance and minimize oral cavity and oropharyngeal dysfunction: speech and swallowing (Fig. 19.10).

Management of laryngeal cancer

Treatment of malignant tumours of the larynx may result in alterations of laryngeal functions – breathing, speech and swallowing. The larynx is oncologically divided into three anatomical subsites – glottis (vocal cords), supraglottis (above the vocal cords) and subglottis.

Early glottic cancer can be effectively treated by endoscopic laser surgery (Fig. 19.11) or by radiotherapy; advanced glottic cancer is treated by chemoradiotherapy or by total laryngectomy (Fig. 19.12). Supraglottic cancers, when small, can be treated by radiotherapy alone and, when the tumour is larger, by partial supraglottic surgery, chemoradiotherapy or total laryngectomy. The neck, either ipsilateral or bilateral, needs to be addressed either by surgery with some form of modified neck dissection, or incorporated into the radiotherapy field of treatment.

Local control by radiotherapy or surgery in early stage glottic cancer should be achieved in 90% or more of patients, with surgical salvage for local recurrence resulting in 95% or more having a 5-year survival. In more advanced glottic cancer, local control of disease by

radiotherapy is 50–70%, with larynx preservation 60%, and overall 5-year survival rates of 60–70%. Supraglottic cancer (Fig. 19.13), because of a higher risk of cervical nodal involvement, has a lower 5-year survival rate than glottic cancers.

Management of hypopharyngeal cancer

Early lesions are usually treated with surgery or radiotherapy. Advanced tumours need both, and chemotherapy may be used as well. As lymph node involvement is usual, tumour resection is usually combined with unilateral or bilateral clearance of neck nodes. The defects in the pharyngeal continuity may need reconstruction with muscle, skin flaps, stomach or free tissue transfer (Fig. 19.14). The prognosis, depending on tumour stage, is from 25 to 80% 5-year survival.

Quality of life

Quality of life issues in head and neck cancer are crucial, given the nature of the disease, stage of presentation and options for treat-

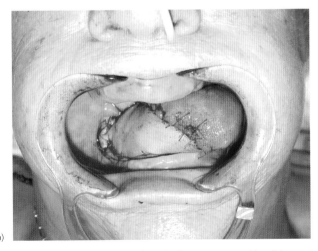
(a)

(b)

Figure 19.10 Surgical resection and repair of tongue cancer: (a) radial forearm free flap and (b) repair of surgical defect (hemiglossectomy).

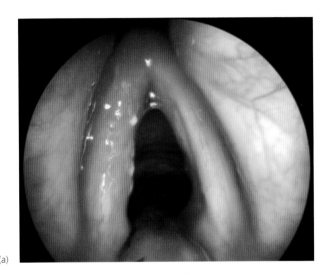
(a)

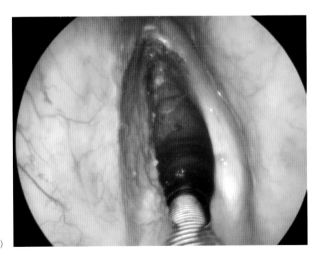
(b)

Figure 19.11 Surgical treatment of early glottic cancer: (a) pre-laser excision and (b) postoperative view.

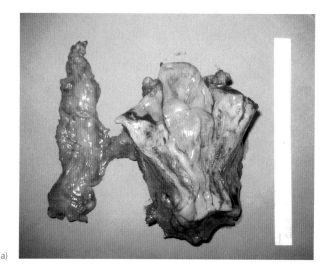

(a)

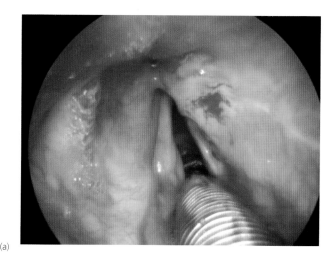

(a)

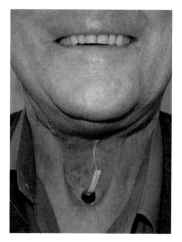

(b)

Figure 19.12 Surgical treatment of advanced laryngeal cancer: (a) total laryngectomy with neck dissection and (b) late postoperative view of tracheostoma with tracheo-oesophageal voice prosthesis (TEP).

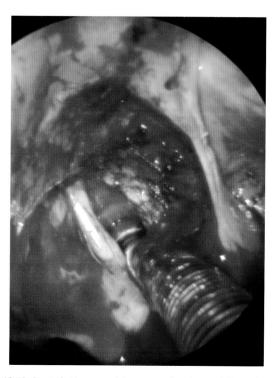

(b)

Figure 19.13 Supraglottic cancer: (a) pre-operative view and)() post-laser excision.

ment and symptom control, which can affect functions such as speech, voice and swallowing as well as facial and cosmetic appearance. These factors have enormous psychosocial effects on the correct decision about treatment, and its long-term effects on life in general. Patients at the time of presentation often have advanced disease, which is currently incurable. They can be helped by the placement of a tracheostomy and/or a gastrostomy tube. Many distressing symptoms can be helped by a short course of irradiation, or chemotherapy. For management considerations, see Box 19.3.

Prognosis

Prognosis depends largely on the stage of disease at the time of presentation, with the single most important factor being the presence of neck node metastases, which reduces the survival by 50%. The presence of more than one node reduces the survival by another 50%. Because of the age and the presence of comorbidities, many head and neck patients die from causes unrelated to their head and neck cancer after treatment. Therefore, management concentrates

on the quality of living and quality of dying. For initial treatment considerations, see Box 19.4.

Box 19.3 **Management goals in head and neck cancer**

- Emphasis on early detection.
- Sound management of pre-cancerous lesions.
- Effective therapeutic measures that are least disabling and disfiguring.
- Early application of measures to achieve maximum feasible rehabilitation.
- Effective palliation for those who cannot be cured.

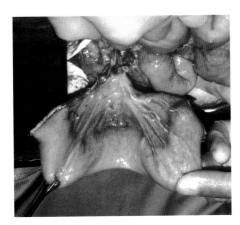

(a)

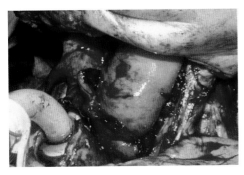

(b)

Figure 19.14 Hypopharyngeal cancer: (a) free jejunal tissue graft and (b) per-operative picture of the graft in position.

Further reading

Alho O-P, Teppo H, Mantyselka P, Kantola S. (2006) Head and neck cancer in primary care: presenting symptoms and the effect of delayed diagnosis of cancer cases. *Canadian Medical Association Journal*; **174**(6): 779–84.

Bradley PJ, Zuchi B, Nutting CM. (2005) Editorial; An audit of clinical resources available for the care of head and neck cancer patients in England. *Clinical Oncology*; **17**: 604–9.

National Institute for Clinical Excellence. *Improving Outcomes in Head and Neck Cancer: Guidance on Cancer Services. The Manual.* National Institute for Clinical Excellence, London www.nice.org.uk

National Institute for Clinical Excellence. *Referral for Suspected Cancer.* National Institute for Clinical Excellence, London, www.nice.org.uk (revised June 2005).

Box 19.4 **Factors determining the choice of initial treatment**

There are three sets of factors to consider.
Patient factors:
- age
- comorbidity
- physiological status
- occupation/lifestyle/socio-economic considerations
- previous treatment.

Tumour factors:
- site
- size
- location – anterior/posterior
- bone involvement
- tumour type
- depth of invasion
- previous treatment.

Physician factors:
- surgery
- radiotherapy
- chemotherapy
- nursing and rehabilitation
- prosthetics
- supportive services.

Report of the National Head and Neck Cancer Audit. www.dahno.com

Scully C, Felix DH. (2005) Oral Medicine: Oral white patches. *British Dental Journal*; **199**: 565–72.

Scully C, Felix DH. (2005) Oral Medicine: Red and pigmented lesions. *British Dental Journal*; **199**: 639–45.

Scully C, Felix DH. (2006) Oral Medicine: Oral cancer. *British Dental Journal*; **200**: 13–17.

Further resources

Cancerbackup, www.cancerbackup.org.uk
Facial Deformity Charity, www.letsface-it.org.uk
Head and Neck Cancer Charity, www.getahead.org.uk
Mouth Cancer Foundation, www.mouthcancerfoundation.org
National Association of Laryngectomy Clubs, www.nalc.ik.com

Index

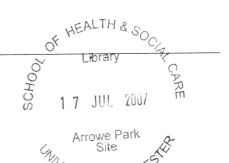